P9-DHD-553

"This book was created for any mom ready to empower herself with effective, natural solutions."
—J. J. Virgin, *New York Times* best-selling author of *The Virgin Diet* and *JJ Virgin's Sugar Impact Diet*

"*Smart Mom's Guide to Essential Oils* is the perfect solution for every mom looking to implement a nontoxic lifestyle."
—Dr. Izabella Wentz, *New York Times* best-selling author of *Hashimoto's Thyroiditis: Lifestyle Interventions for Finding and Treating the Root Cause*

"Dr. Mariza Snyder explains the powerful benefits of essential oils and how to use them in this incredible book."
—Kevin Gianni, best-selling author of *Kale and Coffee: A Renegade's Guide to Health, Happiness, and Longevity* and cofounder of Annmarie Skin Care

"In this practical essential oil guide, Dr. Mariza Snyder teaches you... how to be a smart mom by using effective recipes for overall well-being, green cleaning, personal care, and hormone support."
Dr. Jolene Brighten, ND, best-selling author of *Healing Your Body Naturally After Childbirth: The New Mom's Guide to Navigating the Fourth Trimester*

"Dr. Snyder does a wonderful job in her book guiding moms through all of the essential oil basics for themselves and their families."
—Maya Shetreat-Klein, MD, best-selling author of *The Dirt Cure: Growing Healthy Kids with Food Straight from Soil*

"For those of you new to the world of essential oils, or even if you're a veteran essential oil enthusiast, this book is for you."
—Anthony Youn, MD, America's Holistic Plastic Surgeon™ and best-selling author of *The Age Fix*

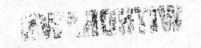

SMART MOM'S GUIDE
TO
Essential Oils

NATURAL SOLUTIONS FOR
A HEALTHY FAMILY, TOXIN-FREE
HOME AND HAPPIER YOU

DR. MARIZA SNYDER

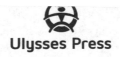

Ulysses Press

Published in the United States by:
Ulysses Press
P.O. Box 3440
Berkeley, CA 94703
www.ulyssespress.com

ISBN: 978-1-61243-646-3
Library of Congress Catalog Number 2016950680

Printed in Canada by Marquis Book Printing
10 9 8 7 6 5 4 3 2 1

Acquisitions editor: Casie Vogel
Managing editor: Claire Chun
Project manager: Serena Lynn
Editor: Renee Rutledge
Proofreader: Shayna Keyles
Indexer: Sayre Van Young
Cover design: Malea Clark-Nicholson
Cover photo: © AmyLv/shutterstock.com
Interior design and layout: what!design @ whatweb.com

Distributed by Publishers Group West

IMPORTANT NOTE TO READERS: This book has been written and published strictly for informational and educational purposes only. It is not intended to serve as medical advice or to be any form of medical treatment. You should always consult with your physician before altering or changing any aspect of your medical treatment. Do not stop or change any prescription medications without the guidance and advice of your physician. Any use of the information in this book is made on the reader's good judgment and is the reader's sole responsibility. This book is not intended to diagnose or treat any medical condition and is not a substitute for a physician.

This book is independently authored and published and no sponsorship or endorsement of this book by, and no affiliation with, any trademarked brands or other products mentioned within is claimed or suggested. All trademarks that appear in ingredient lists and elsewhere in this book belong to their respective owners and are used here for informational purposes only. The author and publisher encourage readers to patronize the quality brands mentioned in this book.

CONTENTS

INTRODUCTION

"Do you want safer, cheaper, more effective natural solutions for you and your family?" I have asked this question to thousands of smart moms across the country while educating them about the benefits of essential oils. Each and every time, I look out at these amazing, loving moms and know that they are ready to embark on their journey toward natural solutions. My sole purpose in creating this book is to empower you, the smart mom, and others around the world with natural solutions that will inspire you and your family to stop waiting around for a wellness solution and take the reins yourself. You can reclaim control over your health and wellness with simple yet powerful lifestyle changes supported by pure, potent, high-quality essential oils!

For years before I started to use essential oils, I leaned a lot on nutrition to keep me and my entire family healthy. Though I believe that nutrition is the foundation to a healthy and vibrant body, essential oils have transformed how we take care of our bodies physically, mentally, and emotionally on a daily basis. Essential oils have become as important as wholesome nutrition in my home and in the homes of millions of families across the world. They bridge the gaps between the foundational lifestyle habits of nutrition, exercise, reducing toxic load, and sleep, and often are the missing link to that hurdle you've been trying to jump.

My first experience with essential oils started with one of my favorites, wild orange. The moment I opened the bottle of this delightful citrus oil, it was love at first smell. The aroma jumped out of the bottle, right through my olfactory bulb and into my limbic brain. Immediately, I felt invigorated with joy and nostalgia for the oranges I ate in my youth. Wild orange quickly became my favorite Energizer Bunny to keep me going during long projects and late nights. I even frequently diffused wild orange and peppermint, one of my go-to pick-me-up blends, while working on this book. I desperately desire to give you the same experience with essential oils.

The moms that I know express true concerns about the effects over-the-counter remedies, cleaning products, and personal care items have on their children. Due to the bombardment of synthetic chemicals right under our noses, adults and children struggle to stay healthy throughout the year. Many of us do not even realize the side effects of the chemicals that show up in nearly every product in our homes. Our children are reacting to these chemicals through skin and gut sensitivities. Luckily, essential oils are revolutionizing the way smart moms and families manage their health. By utilizing the power of essential oils and natural ingredients, many of your everyday products and solutions can be easily and safely made at a significantly lower cost. This is a win-win for everyone!

Over the years, I've learned that navigating the diverse benefits of essential oils can be quite daunting. One of the top concerns of smart moms is how to safely and effectively introduce essential oils into their homes without having to devote hours of study to the process. With over 3,000 identified varieties of aromatic compounds found in essential oils, it can be quite overwhelming for anyone, and the learning curve can be steep if you don't have the right resources in front of you to expedite the process. This guide is my gift to you—the research has been done and the recipes compiled. They are all right here at your fingertips. I truly believe that this book will help you effectively learn about and introduce essential oils to your home while teaching you at a reasonable pace. Before long, your whole house will have gone through an essential oils makeover and will be free of toxic chemicals. You will be amazed at the change you'll see and feel in you and your family's health!

So let's get started! If you are a newbie to essential oils, start by reading Chapters 1 and 2, which dive into those all-important questions about essential oils:

- ❧ What are essential oils and how are they produced?
- ❧ How do you use essential oils safely?
- ❧ How do you store essential oils?
- ❧ How do I dilute them for my children and during pregnancy?

As you dive deeper into this guide, you are going to find natural solutions for everyday family emergencies, from neck tension to digestive upset and much more. If you are looking to revamp your bathroom cabinet and cleaning cabinet, you will find simple, easy-to-make green cleaning and personal care recipes that will revolutionize your routines and improve the health of your family. You are going to love having natural alternatives to synthetic and toxic products! And, even better, you will need fewer products around the house once your essential oil and natural products makeover is complete. Imagine using just one or two products to clean your entire house that smell amazing and are completely safe!

Equally important to physical well-being is mood and emotional balance, and often these play a part in other underlying health issues. How about a way to purify the air in your home while managing moods at the same time? Explore the chapter on aromatherapy and you will be amazed. From simply inhaling their potent aromas to diffusing the oils, the numerous benefits to working with single essential oils or a synergistic blend include balancing the mood and emotional wellness of your household.

We women are powerful CEOs of our families, careers, and communities. We are incredible multitaskers and we make the world go 'round, but we often forget to prioritize ourselves. If we aren't in top condition, everyone around us suffers. Our health is as important as every other priority in our lives. The more on top of our health we can be, the more we can serve others, especially our families and those we love the most. We can also show up bigger, with more energy and joy!

I want to share something with you that it took me a while to realize on my journey: **You are the boss of your healthcare**. You. Not doctors, not nurses, not insurance companies. You. You can create a self-guided action plan toward optimal health for you and your family. Inherently, your body is primed and ripe for healing miracles. By both staying empowered and taking ownership of your health, you can call upon doctors and healers for their expertise, opinions, and support without relinquishing your control. You ultimately have final say in your wellness plan, which should involve a balance of nutrition, exercise, meditation, and/or breathing exercises, and self-care rituals to support and nourish your overall well-being.

The final chapters of this guide explore powerful self-care rituals that you can implement into your daily and weekly schedule. They are designed to help you to reduce stress while increasing your energy and sustaining your vitality. For more targeted support, explore the chapter Women's Hormone Health. As a hormone expert, I recognize the necessity and importance of proper hormonal balance in the body. This is the first step in revolutionizing your family's wellness—taking care of you. There are also recipes and blends to support mood, stress, energy, weight, mental clarity, and libido.

You deserve a body that works for you—we all do! And it's going to take courage to begin to make the changes that put you first when it comes to your health. The first step is deciding that it's time to make some changes. They don't need to be big changes. Start by integrating habits and rituals that will get your body back in balance. Then slowly branch out into some of the other chapters that will help you to make over cleaning, self-care, healthcare, and other routines in your house. Little by little, the change toward natural solutions will begin to happen, and before you realize it, you will have revolutionized the wellness and vitality of your entire family and home! I can't wait for you to join me on this essential journey.

CHAPTER

❧ 1 ❧

WHAT ARE ESSENTIAL OILS?

Scents often elicit memories and emotions from deep within us, no matter how commonplace. From the perky citrus scent of your mom digging into an orange peel while preparing lunches to the comforting scent of fresh rosemary in a homemade chicken soup simmering in the slow cooker, scents tell the story of your everyday life. The foundational aromas of your home not only provide a distinctive olfactory benchmark in your brain, but they also can train your children in daily self-care rituals so that they can attribute scents to solutions for healthcare needs in their adult years. Instilling and practicing self-care rituals in your home today will serve your family in their future healthcare journeys.

Essential oils appear again and again throughout history as a means for perfuming the world and as natural, concentrated solutions for healthcare needs. Not only do certain oils create the distinct aroma of a particular plant, but they also play a role in the plant's survival and participation in the chain of life. The oils within each plant give off a scent to attract or repel various predators or herbivores in order for the plants to multiply. In addition, some plants have an amazing ability to heal themselves when damaged, and the essential oils within play a role in this process. The essential oils found within plants only comprise one to five percent of the plant's total makeup. The amount of plant material needed to produce just one drop of essential oil must not only be carefully grown and harvested, but also gathered in a large quantity to produce the tiniest amount of essential oil.

Essential oils are volatile aromatic compounds located in the bark, stems, leaves, seeds, roots, flowers, and other parts of plants. *Volatile,* in reference to essential oils, means that the tiny organic molecules are able to change states quickly from liquid to gas when at room temperature. In simpler terms, when you twist open a bottle of essential oil, the aroma not only hits you in the face with its scent-packed power, but is also noticeable to someone standing on the other side of the room—or in another part of the house! Both the physical and chemical composition of the essential oil enables it to invade the air it comes in contact with and the olfactory (smell) sensors in the body as you inhale the scent. The uniqueness of each essential oil hinges on the variety of its chemical constituents, which can vary from plant to species. And, with over 3,000 variations having been identified already, that makes for a lot of variety!

Within each essential oil are a variety of chemical constituents, primary and trace, that affect its amazing potent power. Each essential oil can consist of over 800 different constituents, though scientists have only identified 200 of them so far. The myriad influences on a single plant can astound even the most intelligent of scientists, and numerous studies are being carried out each year to discover their impact.

As if there weren't enough nuance in the composition of essential oils, the constituents can also be affected by a number of outside influences, such as when the plant was harvested, from what part of the plant the oil was extracted and by what method, the fertilizer used during the growing season, and the climate, specific weather patterns, and geographic region in which it was grown, to name a few. Even the way the plant is pollinated can affect the composition of the essential oil, altering its constituents and even the scent of the essential oil itself.

This is why it is so important to purchase only the highest quality essential oils from reputable companies who understand that each step in this process is a crucial factor in the end product, and who conduct both independent and in-house quality tests to ensure that they are offering only the best essential oils for you and your family.

Potency of Essential Oils

The super-charged potency of essential oils should always be something that you keep in mind. To create a frame of reference, let's talk numbers for a bit. Essential oils are 50 to 70 percent more potent than their herbal counterparts, meaning that it is a lot more efficient and cost-effective for you to purchase essential oils to use for homeopathic remedies, as well as in everyday cooking, where you might normally use dried herbs. So, what does that percentage mean? Here is a great rule-of-thumb example: one drop of pure, high-quality peppermint essential oil is the same as 28 glasses of peppermint tea. 28 glasses! It may take your mind a while to let that sink in because it is such an amazing fact, but you must fully understand the potency of these oils before using them in your home. We are so used to super-sized life, super-sized portions, super-sized everything that it may take us a moment to step back and realize how far one single drop of essential oil will go and the power that is packed within.

Now let's consider an everyday item used in cooking and flavoring—a lemon. In the grocery store, a lemon may cost anywhere from 50 cents to a dollar, or even more if you are buying organic. We generally use lemons in multiple ways, from juicing for a seafood dish to dropping the rinds in water for a bit of lemon essence as flavoring. Lemons don't seem expensive until you realize how much you might be spending on just lemons in order to create a flavor profile. A bottle of lemon essential oil (EO) usually contains around 250 drops and is one of the least expensive oils to purchase, but there are many, many uses for it. Generally, one drop of lemon EO would cost about four to five cents, but it takes approximately 50 lemons to create a 15-milliliter bottle of lemon EO. The potency of one drop of lemon oil greatly outweighs what you could eke from an entire lemon on your own. Yes, there is something to say for a fresh lemon flavor in cooking, but imagine if you were flavoring your daily smoothie with lemon juice when you could be using one single drop of lemon essential oil! Big difference in cost and in flavor.

Why are some essential oils so incredibly expensive? It usually has to do with the quantity of plant material needed to produce the essential oil. For example, rose essential oil continues to be one of the most costly essential oils on the market. But it takes 105 pounds of rose petals just to make five milliliters of rose essential oil, or 10,000 pounds of petals to distill one pound of rose essential oil! This is why many perfume companies will often substitute a cheaper alternative with chemical constituents that smell similar to a rose in order to keep their costs low. For example, geranium oil has often been used as a substitute for the more expensive rose oil in both the perfume and the essential oil industry. Not only can geranium be subbed for rose oil, but it can also be heavily diluted with a carrier oil, reducing its potency. In the perfume industry, they use "fragrance oils," which are most definitely *not* the same thing as essential oils. In fact, even something touted as "natural fragrance" is most likely a synthetic knock-off.

History of Essential Oils

Imagine being in ancient Mesopotamia over 5,000 years ago, when primitive essential oils tickled the noses and crept into every crevice of life. As an integral part of their rituals and ceremonies, the incense-laced smoke permeated the world of the Mesopotamians as they invoked the spirits to assist them in their healing. Their shimmering bodies pulsed with scent from having anointed themselves with salves made from plants soaked in animal fat or seed oil. Even this long ago, without the distillation process, humans recognized the potency of the plants on this earth and found a way to harness their amazing powers. Truly, they can be credited with harnessing this holistic view of healing mind, body, and soul.

Hopping over to India, we see essential oils as a tool in Ayurveda, a system focused on balancing the energy of a particular body type while maintaining harmony with the word around you through medication, exercise, diet, and lifestyle. Utilizing a massage technique, essential oils are coupled with carriers like coconut or sesame oil for a deep tissue experience of the mind and body. When thinking of Indian aromas, our olfactory lobes instantly trigger musky scents of sandalwood, jasmine, and vetiver, which promote relaxation.

Moving into ancient Egypt, we enter the tombs of mummification, still tingling with the scents of frankincense, cedarwood, spikenard, and myrrh. The hieroglyphics on ancient papyrus document the use of oils in healing various ailments. Archaeologists discovered that King Tut's tomb had been robbed twice: once for precious metals and the second time for embalming salves and cosmetics found in alabaster jars. How amazing is it that these oils were so valued, so prized during this time period that thieves would break into the tomb of a pharaoh just to get their hands on them? And we all know the story of Jesus Christ being brought gifts of frankincense and myrrh by the Wise Men, not to mention numerous other biblical allusions to various oils.

Around the same time, ancient Chinese herbal medicine blossomed, creating one of the most influential medical texts that documented over 300 plants utilized in healing. Noted in their writings were uses for ginseng and the ever-popular citrus oils that we all rely on for our pick-me-ups. The Chinese also believed that a plant's soul could be set free in the extraction of its fragrance.

Hippocrates in Greece wrote about the use of essential oils, and famously used aromatics during the time of the plague in Athens to keep its citizenry from harm. A number of famous Greek physicians have been credited with citing aromatic plants as the key to many health treatments, even though they didn't fully grasp the composition of the essential oils or have a good way to extract these essences. By the time the Romans got a hold of the scents, they were obsessed, scenting everything that could be scented. Add in their fixation on public health, aromatherapeutic baths and massages became a part of their daily lives.

In Arabia, capitalism gave way to more travel for these fragrances. The famous spice trade route introduced frankincense, as well as a variety of other oils, from Omar to Jordan, affectionately known as the Frankincense Trail. The Arabs are also thought to be the first to have used steam distillation as a method for extracting the essential oils. Essential oils then traveled the spice route from Persia to Europe. There, they were famously used to drive the Great Plague out of areas of sickness once it was realized that those people who had aromatics around them were nearly immune to the disease. Fumigations took place daily, with people using the aromatics in a desperate attempt to protect themselves from death.

In the mid-nineteenth century, the popularity of essential oils picked up. During that time, René-Maurice Gattefossé, the "father of aromatherapy," notoriously suffered an accidental burn during his research and treated it with lavender essential oil. Though he knew the oils harnessed powerful healing qualities, he now had firsthand experience with which to relay his findings. Gattefossé coined and studied "aromatherapy" as a healthcare technique, resulting in the book *Gattefossé's Aromatherapy*. While perfumers were focusing on the creation of more synthetic fragrances and medicine was shifting toward synthetic vaccinations and antibiotics, Gattefossé harnessed the healing power he believed to be in the essential oils and made it his life's work to create a compendium of their chemical properties.

In today's world, where antibiotics are no longer as effective as they once were thought to be and where there is a push for more natural methods in healthcare and daily life, essential oils have found a resurgence in popularity in a variety of industries, including scientific study. As we learn more about the chemical composition and constituents of essential oils, scientists are able to recommend alternatives to commonly prescribed medications and over-the-counter treatments. With this popularity comes a need for education in the mainstream population so that everyone is able to utilize the amazing power of these natural oils. Now that some history is under your belt, let's discuss exactly what it is that you are dealing with when you say "essential oils" in today's world.

How Are Essential Oils Produced?

In general, there are four different ways in which essential oils are produced: steam distillation, cold pressing, CO_2 extraction, and solvent extraction. The method chosen depends on several factors, including where the essential oil is located and the potency of oil desired. Intense care must be taken in harvesting the plants before production to ensure that they are not cut, damaged, or changed from their original form in any way. Certain plants need to be altered in order to be placed into the distillation still, usually because the essential oil is contained in a part of the plant not easily accessed.

Steam Distillation

Steam distillation is the most common method by which to obtain essential oils. Basically, the success of steam distillation relies on the fact that essential oils are both volatile and hydrophobic. We all know from basic elementary school science that oil and water do not mix, and the same is true here—essential oils do not mix with water. This hydrophobic nature makes the application of steam ideal for the extraction of essential oils.

Imagine a giant chamber filled with raw, organic plants. In a nearby chamber, water reaches its boiling point. When the steam reaches the required temperature between 140°F and 212°F (60°C and 100°C), depending on the plant material, the steam pushes its way into the bottom of the larger extraction chamber containing the plant material. As the hot steam forces its way up to fill the chamber, the slight pressure created as it passes through the plant material causes microscopic internal sacs that protect the essential oils to burst. Because the molecules are so small, they easily rise out of the main chamber into a condenser, where they are cooled down. As you would expect, the oil and water separate, creating two separate layers: the essential oil and the floral water (hydrosol). Both can then be easily collected for use. (Hydrosol is slightly scented and is often used as an additive in a variety of perfume and beauty products.)

Remember how the uniqueness of each plant requires they be treated with such care in production? The way in which the steam distillation takes place also plays a role in this method. The temperature of the steam, the pressure used, and the time allowed for the process to take place all influence the quality of the essential oil produced. No chemical reaction takes place in this process, just a separation of the compounds. Because of pressurization, the distillation process can take place at temperatures below the boiling points of the oils, which maintains and protects the quality of the essential oils. It also greatly speeds up the processes, allowing for the oils to be distilled in less time but still at a high quality. But, due to the uniqueness of each plant, the time required for distillation varies as well, taking anywhere from a few hours for lavender to a few days in the case of wood oils.

This is yet another reason why I only trust a few essential oil companies, because they pay careful attention to this process to ensure the production of only the purest and most potent essential oils. Preserving the integrity of the essential oil is something that companies like dōTERRA, Young Living, and Rocky Mountain have taken years to perfect and they continue to work on daily to ensure that you are getting the best of the best that they have to offer. For example, dōTERRA performs seven separate quality tests on each and every yield of essential oils to produce their Certified Pure Therapeutic Grade° (CPTG°) essential oils.

Cold Expression (Cold Pressing)

Most commonly used with citrus fruits, cold pressing, or expression, is the method used to extract essential oils from the waxy rinds of fruits without adding heat. You have likely experienced the burst of citrus oils that releases when you peel the rind from an orange or a lemon. To obtain these most volatile of essential oils, the rinds of the citrus fruit are placed in a press. Then, they are simply pressed with mechanical force in order to obtain these uplifting citrus essential oils, or moved back and forth to achieve small cuts that allow the essential oils to be released. Water is then added and the mix is filtered and centrifuged in order to separate the essential oil.

Again, the uniqueness, quality, and potency of the essential oil depends on a variety of factors including exact pressure, harvesting practices, and timing. Only the best artisanal growers are commissioned in partnerships with the companies mentioned above to harvest at the optimum times and utilize a precise distillation process to ensure only the best essential oils that will properly support health and wellness.

Solvent Extraction

For the more delicate plants, such as flowers like jasmine where the essential oils are found in the petals, a careful process of solvent extraction is necessary. The result of this process is not an essential oil, but an *absolute*, which contains both aromatic and non-aromatic chemical constituents. In this process, a solvent is carefully selected to gently wash the petals and dissolve the fragrance-containing compounds. The plant material may need to be broken up or manipulated in order for the solvent to completely penetrate the petals.

Filtering must take place next to separate the larger plant materials left behind, like petals and bark. The remaining substance is vacuum distilled to remove the solvent. This produces what is known as a *concrete*, which contains all the fragrant compounds as well as other fatty compounds. The concrete goes through another solvent processing, usually with an alcohol, to remove the insoluble fatty compounds. A second round of vacuum distillation takes place to remove most of the remaining solvent. Within the remaining absolute, only about one to five percent of the solvent remains. Some aromatherapists are concerned with this remaining amount of solvent, though most consider it to be such a trace amount that there is minimal cause for concern.

CO2 Extraction

CO_2 extraction is a more modern technique where carbon dioxide is used as a solvent in the extraction process. It is a perfect method for use with heat-sensitive oils, since the CO_2 can achieve a state where it is neither gas nor liquid when heated and pressurized. In this state, it is used as a solvent and added to the plant material to release the essential oils. The mixture is then filtered and vacuumed much like in solvent extraction, though in this process, as the CO_2 returns to its normal gaseous state, it evaporates and leaves behind the pure essential oil. Though the equipment is considerably more expensive than in other methods, there is no solvent left behind to worry about, and the CO_2 does not affect the chemical structure or odor of the oil.

How Should I Choose Essential Oils?

Choosing essential oils can be a daunting task, especially for a busy mom. They are popping up all over the place as they increase in popularity, but do not be tempted to pluck one off your grocery store shelf! Yes, it is convenient. But unless you have researched the company and feel comfortable about where and how they are coming by their essential oils, I highly recommend leaving it on the shelf and buying from one of the top companies on the market with trusted practices. A lot of companies are selling highly adulterated oils that will not provide the benefits that you desire, and, honestly, there is no telling what may be in those bottles. There aren't strict regulations for essential oils right now, and this makes it difficult to know exactly what you are getting.

Despite the lax regulations, let's talk about the different grades of oils. It is a well-known fact in the industry that 98 percent of the essential oils produced today are either food- or perfume-grade oils, meaning they are used in food flavorings or perfumes and cosmetics. These oils are heavily adulterated and contain a variety of additives or solvents with the aim of achieving a standard scent, smell, or taste. Imagine if every time you popped the top on your favorite soft drink, you found that it tasted differently! What works for the food industry does not work for the essential oil industry, where they are concerned with the constituents of the oil and the efficacy it will have in terms of healthcare. As a result, most of the oils used in the food and perfume industry are synthetic, chemically engineered oils, because the scent can be standardized and will not vary like different batches of pure essential oils.

Food-grade oils do have several quality standards that they must be met before they can be Generally Recognized As Safe for consumption, or GRAS. All foods that pass the GRAS standard must be stamped with an expiration date. There are essential oils that have passed the GRAS standard and are stamped with expiration dates, but that doesn't mean they are safe to consume or be taken internally as a dietary supplement. Please be sure to consult with your trusted healthcare provider and to do your research before deciding to take oils internally. Personally, I cook with the oils and use them in smoothies and other treats that I make at my house and for my friends. What I don't recommend is ever letting kids or adults with health conditions take drops of pure therapeutic-grade essential oils internally. This is a personal decision that you must make for your family, and one that must be considered carefully.

When dealing with perfume-grade oils, it is generally accepted that about 90 percent of what is sold as a "pure" essential oil in the United States is fragrance grade and diluted. There are several different levels of oil grades, which have most likely been adulterated in addition to being diluted with alcohol and water, and have very few health benefits. In fact, they may even adversely affect your health depending on the colorless, odorless, potentially toxic solvents that may still be lurking in their perfumed oils. Here is a simple chart to help you see the difference:

NAME	% ESSENTIAL OIL	BLENDED WITH	PACKAGING
Eau de cologne	2% to 5% pure	Alcohol and water	Spray/Rollerball
Eau de toilette	4% to 15% pure	Alcohol and water	Spray bottle
Eau de parfum/ Perfume	10% to 20% pure	Alcohol and water	Spray bottle
Perfume	15% to 40% pure	Alcohol	Bottle with stopper

If you are simply looking for essential oils to help to freshen your house or laundry, it may be acceptable to buy something less than therapeutic grade. Heating the oils will break down the precious constituents and make their effectiveness for healthcare a real problem, but if all you want is to have a fresh scent in your warmer to perk up your house, this may not be an issue for you. You may find that using these adulterated oils over time will leave you with a headache or a residue in your warmers, but many people only want the perfume qualities of the essential oils.

A simple test for checking for adulterated oils is the Paper Test: Put a drop of oil on a piece of paper and let it evaporate for about an hour. It should be completely evaporated within this timeframe and should not leave any mark behind. Adulterated essential oils often leave a ring behind from whatever may be lurking in their bottles. This test works for most essential oils except for myrrh and patchouli, and the rare absolutes like rose, jasmine, and vanilla.

When it comes to information about the particulars of essential oils, I always see what renowned chemist Dr. Robert Pappas has to say on the matter. Not only is he thoroughly respected in his field, but a number of companies use his services to third-party test their essential oils. Quality of essential oils is the hot topic today and it is tricky business to navigate through the claims on the shelves. From claims of "pure" to "therapeutic" to "pure therapeutic grade" and even "certified pure therapeutic grade," it is important to understand some basics before you can grasp the details.

If you are in search of the beneficial and awesome power of essential oils, then you should look for therapeutic-grade essential oils. Therapeutic refers to the purity and efficacy of the essential oil's constituents, and, namely, its health benefits. However, another problem is that there is no universal standard for what is known as therapeutic-grade essential oils. Instead, we are left with companies creating their own internal standards and copyrighting their name for it. That is where dōTERRA's Certified Pure Therapeutic Grade® comes from—they perform over seven quality tests throughout the processing of each batch of oil to ensure that it meets their standards for quality, a process that includes paying for third-party testing. Other companies have their own standards, but may not pay for third-party testing. Other companies just plain don't do the testing. This is where it is left up to you, the smart mom, to do a bit of research on your own.

Dr. Pappas asserts, "An oil can be pure...but still be low quality." How is this possible? Simple. Remember the detailed growing, harvesting, and distilling practices that I mentioned before? This is precisely where quality comes into play. You can have a pure oil that was still not grown indigenously, harvested at peak performance time, or distilled with proper care taken with temperature and time. It is a scary prospect, frankly, that there isn't more regulation on the market in this rapidly growing industry, but smart moms need to watch out for their families and not just trust whatever is available on the shelf. Yes, some companies seem to be charging a lot more for essential oils than others, but if these are companies that set their own quality standards and take the time to establish and ensure quality testing in a variety of different areas at numerous points in the production process, then I am more inclined to trust them than some bottles I found on the drugstore shelf.

The best advice I have here is to check out the following:

❀ Does the company source their plants from indigenous regions?

❀ Are the plants harvested at peak times for the highest quality product?

❀ Do they use pesticides on their plants or claim to be organic?

❀ Do they use both gas chromatography and mass spectrometry testing for quality? (Both tests must be used to ensure that the correct compounds are present and that there are no impurities or pesticides present in the final product.)

❀ Do they test for microbial properties, use Fourier transform infrared spectroscopy (FTIR), or do chirality testing? (FTIR testing is performed to ensure the potency and consistent quality of each batch of essential oil through identifying the structural components of essential oil compounds. Chirality testing ensures that no synthetic elements are present in each batch of essential oils tested.)

❀ Is there a process of organoleptic testing? (Organoleptic testing is used as a preliminary quality control test before other tests are conducted. This test involves the use of the human senses—sight, smell, taste, and touch. Expert distillers use their senses as a first line of quality testing to provide immediate clues about the purity of the essential oil.)

❀ Do they work with the people of the countries of plant origin to develop growing partnerships?

❀ Are their business practices and the leaders of their company trustworthy?

Finally, trust your gut. Smell the oil yourself. Is it overbearing or does it smell crystal clean and balanced? Feel the oil in your fingertips. Is it oily or does it leave a residue? Or does it absorb quickly and completely, leaving behind only a clean scent? You can also do a sniff test from a drugstore bottle versus a sample of oil from a respected company. You will be able to smell the difference, guaranteed. And you will only have to use a drop or two of the pure therapeutic-grade oil as compared to many drops of the inferior oil to achieve the same scent or purpose. Do your homework here, mama. It will be worth it for peace of mind!

Judge an Oil by Its Label

When checking out a potential bottle of essential oil, you want to look for a few specifics:

❦ The scientific name of the plants should be clearly labeled on the bottle. If you are buying a diluted oil, the name of the carrier oil should also be listed. If it is a blend of oils, the name of each plant along with its scientific name should be present as well.

❦ Oils should be stored in amber, cobalt, or dark glass bottles fitted with orifice reducers (little plastic inserts that keep out the air). Dropper tops, while convenient, should be added by the consumer after purchasing.

❦ Price should NOT be the same for all of the bottles of oil. A variety of factors come into play for the production of each essential oil, which should dictate a price variance. Oils all priced about the same should be a huge red flag for you!

❦ An expiration date is not a necessity, but it does indicate that the oils may have been approved for use in cooking and it at least gives you an indication as to how long it has been sitting on the shelf.

How Should I Store Essential Oils?

Due to their volatile nature, essential oils must be stored carefully. Remember the four Cs: Cool, Capped, Centered, and Contained.

COOL: Avoid heat and sunlight. Most essential oils come in amber, cobalt, or dark-colored glass bottles to keep them from ultraviolet rays and prevent evaporation from sunlight. Also, take care to avoid heat; if oils are overheated, the chemical composition can break down, thereby losing their efficacy in supporting your healthcare needs. The best place to store them is in a cabinet in a bathroom or kitchen, away from any heating elements.

CAPPED: Keep them tightly capped. Always be sure that the caps on your bottles are screwed on tightly and have orifice reducers in order to prevent evaporation and oxidation.

CENTERED: Keep the bottles upright. The bottles should be kept in an upright position because of their extreme potency and the oil's ability to break down plastic and other materials. Citrus oils are notorious for eating through orifice reducers if the bottle is left tipped and the oil is in contact with the plastic. Most essential oil companies use high-quality plastics (number 1 PETE or number 2 PETE), but you still want to be aware that they can cause erosion over time if left in contact.

CONTAINED: Use only in glass or stainless steel containers. There are certain types of plastic that are resistant to the essential oils and that will not break down as easily, but in general you want to avoid having them come into contact with any sort of plastic. Your best bet is to stick with glass or stainless steel.

The best way to travel with oils or to keep them with you as an on-the-go solution is to find a carrying case. Many companies make keychain kits with elastics to store sample-size bottles for tossing them in a purse, backpack, or suitcase. Larger cases are either padded with foam, if you plan to travel with the full-size versions, or you can acquire a chic wooden box to keep them cool, dark, and upright.

SAFETY TIP: Never leave essential oils where your children can easily get them without permission. It is empowering to teach your kids how to support their own health with essential oils, but you also need to be aware of how often they are using it and in what capacity.

Quick Essential Oil Chemical Property Overview

Having a background in biochemistry, I learned early on that chemistry is the backbone of life here on earth and is inextricably connected to the world around us. When it comes to understanding essential oil chemistry, it's important to know that most essential oils are a complex combination of carbon, oxygen, and hydrogen, with some constituents containing nitrogen and sulfur. Pure essential oils can be subdivided into two specific groups of chemical constituents.

The hydrocarbon group is mostly made up of terpenes (monoterpenes and sesquiterpenes). The oxygenated compounds consist of mostly alcohols, phenols, aldehydes, ketones, esters, and oxides. Here is a brief explanation of each chemical group, along with benefits and essential oil examples.

MONOTERPENES: Common monoterpenes found in essential oils are limonene, pinene, terpinene, and cymene. They cleanse and stimulate mood; contain powerful antioxidants; support digestive, circulatory, and immune function; repel insects, and promote normal cellular growth and vitality.

SESQUITERPENES: Also in the terpene family are sesquiterpenes, which are less prevalent than monoterpenes. Common sesquiterpenes found in essential oils are cedrene, zingiberene, himachalene, and caryophyllene. The main benefits are cleansing, circulation support, digestive support, and the promotion of emotional balance, well-being, and mental clarity.

ALCOHOLS: In the oxygenated compound family, alcohols are among the most valuable functional groups in essential oils. These are groups that are composed of a hydrogen and oxygen atom. Common alcohols found in essential oils are santalol, linalool, and menthol. Main health benefits include cleansing, protecting from environmental threats, calming, improving skin appearance, supporting mood and emotions, and promoting healthy cellular growth.

PHENOLS: Phenols are a very specialized group of essential oil constituents. The chemical structure of phenols lends to powerful antioxidant properties. Phenols are also very potent and can contribute to minor skin irritation. Always dilute oils with a high phenol content. Common phenols found in essential oils are thymol, carvacrol, and eugenol. Main health benefits are protecting from environmental threats, providing powerful antioxidants, and promoting cellular growth.

ALDEHYDES: Aldehydes are typically found in plants in small quantities, but they are known for contributing to the distinct aromas of essential oils. Aldehydes can potentially cause minor skin irritation. It's important to always dilute essential oils that have aldehyde constituents. Common aldehydes found in essential oils are cinnamaldehyde, geranial, and neral. Main health benefits are protecting from environmental threats; calming mood and emotions; supporting healthy digestive, gastrointestinal, cardiovascular, and brain function; and supporting the immune system.

KETONES: Ketones are similar to aldehydes in chemical composition. Common ketones found in essential oils are carvone, camphor, and menthone. Main health benefits include supporting restful sleep; calming mood; promoting mental clarity, healthy digestion, respiratory function; and providing powerful antioxidants.

ESTERS: Esters are formed when there is an esterification reaction between a carboxylic acid and an alcohol group. Common esters found in essential oils are methyl salicylate, linalyl acetate, and neryl acetate. Health benefits include calming mood and emotions, supporting hormones, reducing the appearance of skin blemishes, nourishing the skin, easing muscles tension, and supporting restful sleep.

OXIDES: Oxides are best known for supporting the immune system. Oxides can be recognized based on their proper names, which end with the suffix "-oxide" or "-ol." Common oxides found in essential oils are eucalyptol (also called 1, 8-cineole), rose oxide, linalool oxide, and pinene oxide. Main health benefits include promoting healthy immune function, protecting against environmental threats, supporting healthy respiratory function, promoting mental clarity and open airways, lessening feelings of tension, and promoting vitality.

CHAPTER

❧2❧

HOW TO USE ESSENTIAL OILS

I can't tell you how many times someone I know buys an amazing collection of essential oils and then *just doesn't use them*. Because they are so foreign to many of us, I think we are scared to try something new, so we just go right back to the accepted "pop-an-OTC-pill method" because it is simply what we know. But that doesn't mean that there isn't another way, maybe a better way, to take care of ourselves and our families. In today's world, where organic, green, super-clean, natural ways are sought out and desired, essential oils provide us with an ancient remedy to a new way of living. The naysayers argue that essential oils are so new that they haven't been tested, but they couldn't be more wrong. They have been around for thousands of years and are a common part of many holistic and Eastern methods of healthcare where healing the mind, body, and soul as a unit finds priority over simply masking symptoms so we can function.

Let's start with the basics.

Application Techniques

Three different application methods for essential oils exist, all providing an amazing way for you and your family to experience the remarkable power of essential oils. All of the recipes in this book fall under one of these methods. How you choose to use the oils with your family is entirely a personal decision and one that you should discuss with a trusted healthcare provider before introducing oils into your home. Remember that each person is different and it may take some trial and error to figure out the perfect oil combination for you and your family. Each person may need a different application method for the same oil! With that said, trying out different combinations is part of the fun, so enjoy the experience.

Aromatic

The easiest and most effective way to experience the benefits of essential oils is aromatically, or by aromatherapy. This technique has been used for thousands of years, long before the advanced distillation techniques yielded the essential oils that we know today. Inhaling the powerful aromas of the oils directly and quickly affects your body's olfactory system, with up to 70 percent of the vapors potentially being absorbed into your body. But it doesn't stop there. Amazingly, essential oils have multiple effects on the body by triggering areas of the brain that then stimulate the neurochemistry of other systems.

The super-packed potency of essential oils also applies to their aromas. You can be standing on one side of a room and know when someone has cracked the seal on a bottle of pure eucalyptus oil because the volatile molecules evaporate so quickly into the air. And the more you allow the oil to evaporate into the air, the more intense the aroma and its effect on your systems will be.

There are three main groupings for aromatherapeutic oils: calming/soothing, uplifting, and grounding/balancing. They are grouped this way due to their primary chemical constituents, which trigger specific emotional responses. For example, floral aromas fall into the calming category due to their primary ester and alcohol composition, while citrus oils are rich with uplifting monoterpenes such as limonene and beta-pinene. You will see me use the terms calming, soothing, uplifting, grounding, and balancing to describe the different oils that I recommend throughout the book.

How do I go about inhaling the oils?

There are a variety of ways to inhale the oils, from simply cracking the top and inhaling deeply from the bottle to using an electronic diffuser. Each has its own benefits, and I recommend employing all the different methods to see what works best for you and your family. Personally, I use essential oils in a variety of ways every day and encourage you to do the same.

Direct inhalation is the simplest method of introducing the oils to your system to affect your emotions or your mood. All you have to do is hold an open bottle or vial near your nose and inhale. Be careful how close you put the oils to your nose and eyes, however, because some are very potent. It is always best to proceed with caution until you know how an oil affects you. Direct inhalation is the first boundary line to cross when introducing a new oil into your repertoire.

With each inhale, the microparticles of the oils are drawn deeper into your system, moving from your respiratory receptors into the olfactory system of your brain. From there, they trigger the limbic system, which can directly affect a variety of functions like emotions, memory, and sleep. The microparticles also take a trip through your respiratory system, where they are absorbed into your lung tissues. This can greatly support your respiratory health. They also hop into your bloodstream and take the incredible journey through your entire body, doing their magic along the way through each vein and internal organ. Eventually they are evacuated via the kidneys, lungs, and pores, but not before going where they are needed and helping to support a variety of bodily systems, especially the hormone-balancing endocrine system.

The next step is to put a drop or two of oil in your palms, rub them together, and then create a cup with your hands and bring it in front of your mouth and nose. You don't want to touch your face with your hands if you haven't yet patch-tested the oil on your skin, but just breathe in the aroma deeply.

Indirect inhalation involves putting drops of essential oil on a vessel, which will then release its aroma into the air. Some people use cotton balls or pads, handkerchiefs, or even tissues that they can then place in strategic locations around their house for a variety of needs. This is also a great way to use aromatherapy in your car, your gym bag, or other small places. Taping a cotton ball to your ceiling fan or air vents in your house or car can really affect the air in a room or small space. Even a drop of oil on the inside of the toilet paper tube will give you a burst of aroma with every roll! A drop of lavender essential oil on a pillowcase or mattress after changing sheets, or on a stuffed animal or blanket, will promote a restful night's sleep. Another tip is to put a drop or two on your air-conditioning filters to release the aroma throughout your house. There are actually a number of hospitals that are now using essential oils in their ventilation systems.

Steamers or *hot water vapor* are another way to work some aromatherapy magic, though the heat may reduce some of the effectiveness of the oil. A steamer is simply a mug of water hot enough to release steam with essential oils added to it. You can simply breathe it in by sitting it in front of you, or you can create a tent with a towel over your head for a more intensified effect. Hot water vapor can also help to work the aroma through the air and into your body. Many people find that placing a cotton ball with a drop or two of oil in the shower with them releases a powerful aroma. You can also make shower bombs that dissolve as you bathe and release aroma.

Diffusion or *nebulizing diffusion* creates a fine mist from the essential oils that are then airborne and pervade an entire area. There are special diffusers made for this process. It is recommended that you only diffuse for 15 to 30 minutes at a time and then take a 45- to 60-minute break to allow your olfactory system to recover; otherwise, the effects of the oil may be diminished. Always check the specific oil that you plan to diffuse to be sure that it is safe for everyone in your family. Diffusing essential oils can be especially beneficial for anyone in your family that requires extra respiratory support; however, be sure to thoroughly discuss and formulate a plan with your healthcare provider, especially if you have been using a humidifier in the past.

For the most effective diffusion, choose an *ultrasonic cool-air diffuser*. It uses ultrasonic vibrations to convert oil mixed with water into a fine water vapor, causing the oils to remain suspended in the air for several hours. This oxygenates the molecules of the air and improves the quality of the air you are breathing, allowing you to safely breathe in the oils, which are then dispersed through your body. Always follow the manufacturer's directions that come with your diffuser to ensure that you are using the correct amounts of water and essential oil. Take the quality of the essential oil that you are using into consideration as well. A diffuser-and-essential-oil combo bought at a supermarket or thrift mass retailer will not be the same quality as a pure therapeutic grade essential oil purchased from a trusted company. To ensure you are receiving the most benefit from your diffuser, make sure to use a pure therapeutic-grade essential oil.

There are some amazing ultrasonic cool-air diffusers available on the market today, especially those with alternating zen light features. These are perfect for use in your kids' rooms, especially if they are comforted by nightlights and a soft hum when they are going to bed. The combination of the appropriate essential oil for their needs and the diffuser will help to support a restful night's sleep, or even keep them focused and centered while doing homework or a project. Diffusers are a necessary tool for any family. And just think—there is a way to get essential oils to your entire family without having to tackle each member and apply the oils individually. Bonus for any smart mom!

A *cool-air nebulizing diffuser* is another option, although more costly, that converts the essential oils directly into the room temperature air without the need for water or any water vapor or mist. The essential oil bottle is typically attached directly to the diffuser and operates on timed intervals. It is great at dispersing the oils over a wide area, typically covering hundreds of square feet in seconds.

Other options include diffusers that blow air through a pad soaked with a few drops of essential oils. This works, but not as well as the other options. Any diffuser that recommends a heating element or source that comes in contact with the essential oils should not be used, as the heat breaks down the constituents of the essential oils, making them less effective for therapeutic benefits. If all you are after is a scent, then it can be effective, but you are better off buying something specifically for aroma without therapeutic qualities.

Humidifiers and *vaporizers* can be used but are not recommended. Your best bet will always be a diffuser. Never put essential oils into a humidifier's water reservoir, as the oils can break down the plastic and leach toxins into the air as the device pushes out the contaminated steam. The best method, if this is what you have at home, is to apply a few drops of essential oils to a cloth or tissue and then place this in front of the air intake area so that the aroma will be pulled through and emitted through the output. Even if the humidifier manufacturer says that it would be okay to use essential oils with its product, it is most likely referring to its own recommended product or something that is highly diluted or adulterated, and it most likely recommends sporadic use and frequent cleaning or filter changes.

Topical

Topical, or direct, application is simply applying the oils right where they are needed on the skin for a direct effect. The microparticles of the oil are able to mix with the natural sebum of your skin and be absorbed into the body. They move into the lymphatic system and then into the soft tissue, where they affect your muscles and all their connective and surrounding tissues. Eventually, they enter the bloodstream and move through the organs before being evacuated, but not before providing invaluable support to your bodily systems. Remember that essential oils are extremely potent, so you only want to use one drop (if that!) at a time for topical applications. You also always want to dilute the oils with a carrier oil, like coconut, jojoba, sweet almond, or grape-seed oil, when using them with children or on sensitive skin. Topical application provides a dual effect to your system; while your skin is slowly absorbing the oils, your olfactory system is getting a quick aromatherapeutic benefit as well.

How do I apply it?

With pure, high-quality essential oils, we always talk in terms of drops. In general, you simply put a drop in your hand or on your fingertip and apply directly to the desired or needed area. There are two terms that you need to know when discussing application: neat and diluted.

Neat means applying the oil directly from the bottle. As mentioned above, this is not recommended for infants or young children, and there are only certain oils that can be applied safely neat, such as frankincense and lavender. However, it is always recommended to dilute all essential oils and then increase the concentration if needed.

Diluted means adding a carrier oil to the essential oil in order to decrease the potency. It essentially allows you to apply less oil for the same effect. Our skin may not respond well to neat application of certain essential oils because they are so potent and drying. The carrier oil allows for a more efficient absorption of the oil on a greater surface area of skin. Research has indicated that diluting essential oils does not decrease their efficacy, but actually enables the oils to be absorbed better because dilution keeps the volatile oils from evaporating too fast. Because essential oils are lipophilic, meaning both attracted to and soluble in fatty substances like carrier oils, the dilution process creates a number of benefits, such as improved absorption.

There are certain oils that are skin sensitive for all people and always require dilution. For example, some essential oils like oregano and clove are known as *hot oils*, meaning that they create a heat sensation and often a burning effect. Others are called *cooling oils*, like peppermint, and cause a cooling or tingling sensation on the skin. See the chart on page 35 for more on hot and cool oils.

Carrier oils are fatty vegetable, nut, or seed oils that blend well with essential oils in order to dilute them. The most commonly used carrier oil is fractionated coconut oil. Raw coconut oil is a white semi-solid at room temperature, much like vegetable shortening, but when heated, it becomes a clear liquid. Fractionated coconut oil is a form that is always clear liquid at room temperature. You want to make sure that you are choosing organic, cold-pressed coconut oil for both raw and fractionated. With raw coconut oil, you have two choices, refined or unrefined, which basically refers to whether you want an almost scent-free version or one that has the coconutty, beachy smell that we love in the summer. Most people choose refined so that the scent of the oils are uncompromised, because sometimes that coconut goodness can either overpower or greatly change the main essential oil component that you are going for. It is a personal choice, really, but I would stick with raw organic cold-pressed refined coconut oil.

Another great choice is jojoba oil, since it very closely resembles the oil our skin produces naturally (sebum), and because of its long shelf life. I often opt for jojoba when making creams or salves for the face, since the skin there is different from that of other areas of the body. Two other options are those that have shorter shelf lives than the others: sweet almond oil and grape-seed oil. Sweet almond oil has a light scent and slight almond color, but works well as a carrier for most blends and is rich with vitamins B and E. If you are allergic to any tree nuts, I would avoid using sweet almond oil. Grape-seed oil is very light with a greenish tint and a slightly nutty smell. Most people use it for massage oil blends. Be sure to choose expeller-pressed instead of solvent-extracted versions of theses oils to avoid any extra chemical elements.

SAFETY TIP: Don't ever try to wash off essential oils with water! Oil and water do NOT mix. The application of water will simply push the oil deeper into your system. Always, always dilute with a carrier oil, or even plain vegetable oil or olive oil from the kitchen; any kind will do to dilute the potency of the oil. This is very important to know with kiddos in the house, especially when using the oils on the kids for the first time.

Where do I apply essential oils?

The general rule of thumb is to always apply the oil either directly to the problem area or as close to it as you can get. For example, let's say your preteen plays outside all afternoon and forgot to ask for you to spritz on some all-natural bug spray. She winds up with several mosquito bites, some on her legs and a nice doozy of a bite right on her eyelid. For the leg bites, you would be okay applying some diluted lavender oil directly to the bites. For her eyelid, though, you will want to both dilute the oil and apply it somewhere near the bite, but not directly on her eye. I would recommend on the temple, or behind the ear closest to the bite. The oils will go where they are needed.

PULSE POINTS: Pulse points are exactly what they sound like—parts of your body where you can take your pulse. Your neck, your wrists, over your heart, and even down by your ankles are all great places to apply oils. They will not only absorb into your skin and help your body from the inside out, but you will also be left with an aroma that will provide an amazing aromatherapeutic experience for you that will last much longer than any perfume or cologne.

FEW SPOTS: Feet, ears, and wrists are the places on your body that have the largest pores. Because of this, the FEW spots are the best places to apply oils when you want a quick absorption rate. The feet especially are like a pipeline to the body, and you can couple this with a reflexology chart to find the exact location on the feet to apply certain oils for maximum efficacy. For example, if your darling daughter is in the throes of a sinus infection, you can massage some cardamom essential oil right into the pads of her toes for respiratory support. (There are also reflexology charts for the ears as well!)

WHERE NEEDED: The best place to apply the oils is always directly (or close to) where they are needed. For example, if you need some respiratory support, apply the oils directly to your chest. You then get the benefit of the oils being absorbed right into your lung tissue while also getting the inhaled reaction. To intensify this effect, you can create what is called a "T-shirt tent," where you simply tuck your mouth and nose down inside the collar of your T-shirt and inhale a few deep breaths, and then release. To push the oils deeper into an area of need, you can also add a wet, warm compress. The water repels the oil, and it is then pushed deeper into your skin until it reaches the target area.

LAYERING: Oils can also be applied one on top of one another in a systematic way known as layering. You simply apply the first oil, rub it in, and then apply the next oil directly on top of the first, repeating the process until you have finished. You only have to wait a few seconds in between each application. Certain oils, such as peppermint oils, are known as driver oils and should always be applied last, since they "drive" the other oils deeper into your system.

Can I use essential oils with massage?

We all love a good rubdown, and this is often a good way to get your partner involved! When applying the oils to a large area of the body, it is important to use a carrier oil that will not only dilute the oil but will also enable you to work it into a greater area for a quicker overall benefit. A good massage dilution rate is 15 to 30 percent, which would be about a 1:3 ratio, or 1 drop of essential oil for every 3 drops of carrier oil. Unless you are a certified massage therapist, I recommend only using gentle strokes and pressure when using the oils, and avoid any sensitive areas. Never give a massage to pregnant women, babies, young children, or anyone with a health condition without first consulting a trusted healthcare provider. Be sure to see the recommended dilution chart on page 36.

Reflexology

Reflexology charts have long been used in a variety of healthcare and holistic settings. By consulting a reflexology chart, you can pinpoint a safer area of application for essential oils that will target an area of need. For example, if your son frequently deals with constipation but has sensitive skin on his belly, you can try applying diluted fennel essential oil to the middle of the arch on his feet, the area indicated for colon support, and massage it in a circular motion. A secondary point would be the inside of his shin from his knee to his ankle. Following application, pull on a pair of baseball socks and let the oils do their work! Reflexology works on several areas of the body, including the hands, feet, and ears. Again, always check with a trusted healthcare provider before using a new essential oil application method on your kiddos or yourself.

Baths

Essential oil baths are an amazing way to experience the effects of the oils throughout your entire body, coupled with the aromatherapeutic benefit. Just remember that hot water not only opens up your pores, enabling the oils to penetrate your system more quickly, but it also can reduce the efficacy of the oils. Never simply drop essential oils into your bathwater or they will just float on the surface. Always add one-quarter cup of Epsom salt to a tub of *warm* water before adding no more than three to six drops of essential oils and swirling the bathwater before you sink in. I would not recommend soaking for more than 20 minutes in an essential oil bath.

Be sure to check out the amazing recipes for shower gel, bath salts, and body sprays in Chapter 6.

Compresses

There are times when oil-and-water repulsion comes in handy, such as when you have deep muscle aches or need respiratory support due to congestion or other issues. This method has proven to be very effective in pushing the oils directly and deeply to the area that most needs support. Using recommended essential oils for your need, you can massage in the oils and then amplify the effects by applying a warm compress, such as a warm washcloth. This will again have multiple benefits, as the warm compress will open up your pores, the slight steam effect will create an aromatherapeutic benefit, and the water will force the oils deep into the area of need. You can also use cool compresses for soothing tension or heat, or for supporting bruises, swelling, or sprains.

Internal

Internal usage of essential oils is a hot topic. Some recommend it, some don't, some strictly forbid it, and most of us are just left confused. The best advice I can give you here is to do your smart mom research and make a personal decision for you and your family. I would never recommend internal usage for children under the age of six, pregnant women, or those with serious health conditions without first consulting a trusted healthcare provider. However, I do personally use them in my cooking as well as take them internally daily as a health supplement. This is only after finding a company that I completely trust and support, and after doing a *lot* of research as to the science behind essential oils and internal consumption. I know a lot of mamas who cook with essential oils for their families, even with kids under the age of six, but they aren't having them take pure, undiluted oils as supplements. Because this is such a touchy area, I will leave it up to you to make your decision. You can always check out my blog for more amazing essential oil recipes for you and your family!

Safety Tips and Precautions

Always, always discuss using essential oils with a trusted healthcare provider before jumping into them full force. Only you and your healthcare provider can make the decision that is right for you and your family. It is especially important to discuss essential oil use if you take any medications or you have any medical conditions.

Most reactions or sensitivities occur because an oil has not been diluted enough. A plant protein needs to be present in order for an allergic reaction to occur, and most of the proteins are removed during the distillation process with essential oils. The proteins present on your skin may react with the essential oil and cause a reaction, but generally if you have diluted the oil enough, you should be fine. Still, if you are terribly allergic to a certain plant or flower or spice, you should use extreme caution when working with essential oils. You must understand that even if you do not apply the oils directly to your skin but instead use an aromatherapeutic approach, your body still may have some sort of negative reaction to the scent. The oils affect your body at a systemic level and even smelling the oils can cause a reaction, just like smelling a food you dislike or a skunk's odor can make you nauseous.

Patch testing is the best way to check for any sensitivities or reactions to essential oils. It is an easy process. Simply add one drop of essential oil to one teaspoon of carrier oil and rub it on a small area of your body. I always suggest that people patch test in more than one location for kiddos as well. The best place to start is the bottoms of the feet and wait 24 hours. Then move on to the area where you intend to apply the oil. Where kids are concerned, you may find that there is some sensitivity on other places of the body but not on the bottoms of the feet. You may also discover that a greater dilution will not cause a reaction, so don't write off an oil over one skin reaction. If you do have a reaction to the essential oil, remember *not* to wash it off with water, because the water will only push the oil in deeper. Dilute the area with more carrier oil over the next few hours until the area of irritation is gone, and be sure to contact your healthcare provider if you have any lingering concerns over the reaction.

Phototoxicity, or photosensitivity, is a concern when using citrus and other essential oils. For at least 12 to 72 hours after application, citrus oils and other phototoxic oils can cause a horrible reaction on the skin, resulting in a mild effect like hyperpigmentation (darkening of the skin) to more serious effects like first, second, and third degree burns. Take care not to use phototoxic oils on exposed skin, especially in the summertime, or at any time when your skin will be exposed to direct sunlight and UV rays. Some of the most phototoxic oils include lemon, lime, wild orange, grapefruit, bergamot (one of the worst for phototoxicity), and most cold-pressed citrus oils. This applies to regular citrus fruit juice during the summer as well, moms. We all love a little lemon juice to lighten our hair in the summer, but imagine that effect on your kiddos' skin. Don't let your kids suck on lemons or limes in the summer time or any time they will be out in the direct sunlight, and be sure to wipe off their sweet faces after drinking fresh-squeezed lemon or limeade of any kind. Here are some potentially phototoxic oils:

Angelica	Grapefruit
Anise	Lemon
Bergamot	Lemon verbena
Bitter orange	Lime
Celery/celery leaf or seed	Mandarin orange
Coriander	Orange
Cumin	Tagetes
Dill	Tangerine
Fig leaf absolute	Wild orange
Ginger	Yuzu

Skin-sensitive oils are another category where you want to be careful. Certain oils, like peppermint and wintergreen, are known as cooling oils due to their cooling effects on the skin. Other oils are known as hot oils for their warming and even burning effects on the skin, such as clove, oregano, cinnamon, or cassia. Often, oils will have a warming sensation on your skin, especially among those who have sensitive skin naturally. Just be aware of this and always start by diluting oils first. Dilution is key when it comes to using these oils, and you always want to be careful not to cross-contaminate from one body part to the next when using these oils. For example, don't touch your eyes or inside of your nose after the application of one of these oils.

SKIN-SENSITIVE HOT OILS	SKIN-SENSITIVE COOLING OILS
Cassia	Camphor
Cinnamon	Eucalyptus
Cinnamon bark	Lemongrass
Clove	Ocotea
Hyssop	Peppermint
Oregano	Spearmint
	Thyme
	Wintergreen

Dilution and Kids

Always dilute oils when using them with kids. Their skin is very different from an adult's, as is their entire systemic makeup. We cannot treat them like little adults, because they just aren't. Their little bodies must be treated with tender care, and using essential oils is something that can work when done correctly and with caution. Only introduce one oil at a time and wait at least 24 hours before reapplying.

I know some moms who follow the same rule with essential oils that they do with new foods—only one new thing per week until they are sure that it doesn't cause any sensitivity or reaction. And just like introducing new foods to babies, dilution is key. We thin out the baby food with breast milk, formula, or even water to make it easier for a baby to digest because their tiny tummies just aren't ready for the full-blown food proteins. In the same way, we dilute the oils because children's bodies aren't capable of handling neat application, and research has shown that they benefit more from the dilution process.

Unless otherwise advised by your healthcare provider, avoid using eucalyptus, peppermint, rosemary, and wintergreen around babies and young children because menthol and other constituents can potentially slow or stop breathing, especially in those with respiratory issues.

For children younger than the age of three months, I do *not* recommend using any essential oils. Their skin is simply not mature enough to handle it. You can use coconut oil as a diaper cream or body lotion, but hold off on essential oils. Again, this is also something to discuss with your trusted healthcare provider. If your little one is a preemie, you want to err on the side of caution and go three months from their due date, not their actual birthdate, when introducing essential oils.

After kids hit the three-month benchmark, I would only start with very mild oils heavily diluted in a mild carrier like coconut oil. A one percent dilution is the best place to start, which is one drop of oil in about 10 milliliters of carrier oil. Lavender is a great oil to start with for babies, as it supports restful sleep and can help ease the tension associated with gas or teething. Other oils to introduce include Roman chamomile, lemon, frankincense, melaleuca, and wild orange. (Do remember that many citrus oils are phototoxic, however.)

At six months, I still recommend a high dilution rate of one to two percent for most oils, but you can branch out a little bit more in terms of which oils you are using. You can begin to introduce a wider variety based on the needs of your little one and the advice of your healthcare team. Oils that should be safe at this age include cardamom, cypress,

ESSENTIAL OIL DILUTION CHART FOR KIDS
(essential oils are not recommended before the age of 3 months)

AGE	DILUTION	DROPS OF EO PER 10 ML CARRIER OIL
3 to 6 months	1%	2 drops
6 months to 1 year	1% to 2%	2 to 4 drops
1 to 5 years	2%	4 drops
5 to 11 years	5%	10 drops
11 to 17 years	10%	20 drops
17+ years	10% to 25%	20 to 50 drops

geranium, ginger, marjoram, rosemary, sandalwood, thyme, and ylang ylang.

Once they hit the toddler age of one year, you can use two drops to 10 milliliters of a carrier oil. Use the dilution chart on page 36 as a guide for older kids. In general, you can add a few more drops to increase the dilution percentage as kids age, but you still want to pay attention to how your child reacts to each oil. Patch testing in advance is always a great way to be sure that there will not be any reactions to the oils.

Just as you would with yourself, you want to avoid applying the oils anywhere close to the mucous membranes on the face, the eyes, the inner ears, in or on the genitals, and directly on broken or damaged skin. You can use essential oils in a diaper cream, but do not insert it vaginally. Be sure to never leave the oils out where kiddos can get a hold of them and do not ever let an infant suck on an oil bottle or rollerball bottle. If the oils do get into an undesirable area, remember to *always dilute* with a carrier oil (even vegetable oil) and then wipe it off. Never, never attempt to wash it off with water. The water will only drive the oil in deeper and cause more harm.

Oils and Pregnancy (and Beyond)

If you are a pregnant or nursing mama, you definitely want to discuss using essential oils with your midwife or OB/GYN as well as your lactation consultant. There are lots of differing opinions out there for moms who want to use oils. I know mamas who used them during childbirth but stopped immediately afterward, mamas who used them all the way through their pregnancy and beyond, and mamas who didn't use them at all throughout their pregnancy and waited until their baby hit three months. It is a personal decision for you to make with your healthcare team.

That said, there is a short and a long answer to the question, "Which oils are safe during pregnancy?" According to trusted midwife Stephanie Fritz, you want to avoid clary sage or sage until you are in labor. While nursing, peppermint has caused a decreased milk supply in some women, so most ladies opt to avoid it entirely while breastfeeding. After that, there are definitely a number of lists floating around as to what to avoid, but it is a decision that you must make for yourself with the help of your healthcare team.

Here is a list of oils to **avoid** during and surrounding pregnancy:

Angelica

Aniseed

Basil

Birch

Black pepper

Camphor

Cassia

Chamomile

Cinnamon

Clary sage (Unless you are in labor. Talk to your midwife or doctor.)

Clove

Fir

Horseradish (typically undesirable oil)

Hyssop

Idaho tansy

Jasmine

Juniper

Marjoram

Mugwort (typically undesirable oil)

Mustard

Myrrh

Nutmeg

Oregano

Pennyroyal

Rosemary

Sage (unless you are in labor)

Thyme

Wintergreen

Oil usage depends on the trimester you are in as well. For safety, there are different guidelines for all three trimesters. Application methods also vary. Any preexisting health conditions or issues with your pregnancy that you may have, any medications that you are on or may need to take, the functioning of your systems while pregnant (such as blood pressure or blood sugar readings), and your sensitivity to the oils (which may change during pregnancy) are all considerations that you should discuss with your healthcare team. Our bodies go through so many changes while we are growing a human being inside of us, which is an amazingly beautiful and immense task. You must adapt your whole world to your newly pregnant and ever-changing body during these nine months and beyond.

In addition to consulting with your team of healthcare professionals, tap into your mother's intuition when making the decision. Only you can decide what is best for you.

The following essential oils are generally considered **safe** during pregnancy:

Geranium

Grapefruit

Lavender

Roman chamomile

Ylang ylang

Lavender, roman chamomile, and ylang ylang essential oils provide a calming mood during stressful moments and encourage restful sleep. I recommend adding one drop of each to a diffuser, or diluting them and applying to the bottom of feet before bed or during times of stress.

Geranium is wonderful for promoting healthy skin during pregnancy, and the floral scent can be energizing during moments of low energy.

Grapefruit can be used for occasional nausea by applying 1 drop to the palms and taking 2 to 3 deep belly breaths. Grapefruit can also be energizing.

First Trimester

During the first trimester, your body is in a very delicate condition while it works overtime to develop that tiny embryo. Exhaustion will hit, morning sickness may take over, and as your stomach expands, you will discover a whole list of symptoms that you may have never dealt with before like gas, bloating, skin issues, and muscle cramps. I would recommend only inhaling the aroma of certain oils to cut morning sickness during the first trimester; topical applications should be extremely limited. Citrus oils with a tart, tangy scent seem to help a lot of women, so sniffing some lemon, lime, or grapefruit may help cut that nausea. On the other hand, some women find that mint helps, so sniffing some peppermint every now and then may be the key for you. Ginger essential oil may also help ease the nausea when inhaled or extremely diluted and applied topically at the end of the first trimester. Near the end of your first trimester, your breasts may begin to feel tender and sore in preparation for breastfeeding, especially your nipples.

Heavily diluted lavender, geranium, or Roman chamomile can help to soothe the ladies. Coconut oil, sweet almond oil, or grape-seed oil are recommended carrier oils.

Second Trimester

One you hit your second trimester, the baby has passed many developmental milestones. At this time, very heavily diluted essential oils are utilized by many midwives. Cardamom, fennel, and ginger are often recommended for indigestion, gas, bloating, or constipation. Helichrysum and frankincense can be diluted and spread over the stomach in areas where stretch marks may appear. Massaging coconut oil into your nipples will also help to prepare them for breastfeeding. And sleep, which you so desperately need, can be greatly supported by diffusing lavender or ylang ylang and massaging it into pulse points and on the top of your feet. A great foot massage or an Epsom salt bath with lavender or ylang ylang before bedtime can be a real asset.

Third Trimester

Once the third trimester takes over, you can relax a bit about the use of essential oils and move into survival mode until your beautiful baby comes along. Continue to use the oils recommended above for heartburn, gas, and bloating as your belly begins to take over all of the room in your body. Massaging the perineum with a coconut oil and frankincense or geranium rub will greatly aid that area during childbirth and support your immune system in the process. Lavender will become your best friend for sleep support in those rocky last months. If you experience issues with respiratory health due to decreased room in your body, diffusing cardamom or eucalyptus may help to promote healthy lung function.

Labor and Delivery

During labor and delivery, essential oils can be your best friend. Be sure to discuss this with your healthcare provider in advance and with the place you will be delivering to see if they have any concerns about essential oil usage. I would definitely add essential oils to your birth plan so that it is clear what your preferences are (though you may change your mind when the time comes!). Diffusing lavender can not only help to calm you during this emotional time, but it will also calm everyone else in the room. You can also apply diluted lavender topically to areas of need. Some women like to be touched and caressed during labor, so a lavender massage can help. Applying diluted clary sage topically to your hips, the bottoms of your feet, and directly on your abdomen will help to promote uterine contractions and ease labor along. During transition, applying one to two drops of diluted basil to your temples and abdomen can also promote labor. Helichrysum is also an amazing essential oil to use to support your menstrual healing and any postpartum bleeding.

While Nursing and Beyond

Nursing mamas have found that many essential oils can help them heal after delivery and can also promote milk production. Lavender will still be your best friend for calming and supporting your mood. To prevent postpartum depression, I recommend diffusing calming and uplifting oils such as lavender and grapefruit while you are alone; oils diffusing around the tiniest babies is not a good idea. You can apply diluted clary sage and lavender topically to your temples or forehead to help with your mood and balance hormones; you can also create an Epsom salt bath for yourself with these oils.

For stretch marks and other skin issues, and for recovery from a C-section, essential oils can also be extremely helpful. Diluted lavender can be a true benefit to this area, as well as myrrh essential oil. Plus, you will get the benefit of the calming properties of these oils as you apply them directly to your areas of concern.

Nursing mamas can find support with a variety of essential oils that support milk production. Diluted clary sage can help to jump-start your milk production and can be applied anywhere on the body. Remember that you don't want to get the oils on your baby's skin, so apply in areas where they will not be immediately touching. Diluted fennel and basil also help to increase the production of milk if you find that you don't have enough. You can apply these directly to the breasts after a feeding when your baby won't be in direct contact with your skin, but do not use fennel for more than 10 days in a row as it may affect your urinary tract system. If you have issues with mastitis during nursing, diluted lavender with a warm compress can help to ease the discomfort. When the time comes that you are ready to wean, diluted peppermint essential oil can help to stop the production of milk when applied topically. It should be avoided during your nursing period for this reason.

Once your baby is over three months of age, you can begin to introduce essential oils one by one into their daily life to help support their immune system and promote healthy growth. Be sure to discuss essential oil usage with your baby's pediatrician in order to develop a safe and effective plan for their health.

CHAPTER

❧ 3 ❧

THE VALUE OF DAILY USAGE

One of the most valuable things that you can do for your family is to incorporate essential oils into a daily healthcare routine. From diffusing to topical application to using them in your cleaning and home-care products, essential oils provide an amazing aroma and therapeutic benefit while they work to affect mood and stabilize your living environment in a natural, nontoxic way. Consistent oil usage is the key to finding the balance that you seek. Researching and learning more about the variety of essential oils available to you will only improve your understanding of how you and your family tolerate individual oils, which application methods are most effective, and what works for your routine.

While completely making over your everyday routines to incorporate essential oils may seem like a daunting task, the truth is that it will happen before you know it. Day by day, as you begin to phase out the old chemical toxins and replace them with the smart recipes in this book, you will be establishing a daily routine of oil usage for your family before you even know what happened. Before long, you will wake up and take an invigorating shower with your homemade peppermint and wild orange body wash, then shave your legs with the shaving cream that you just made and enjoy that you won't have to moisturize afterward because of the coconut-shea-jojoba combo with the grapefruit essential oil kicker. Brushing your teeth with your homemade toothpaste, you will enjoy the fresh kick of peppermint and know that your oral hygiene is not the only benefit your body is getting from that essential oil. Dabbing on some of your newly blended rollerball of grounding essential oil perfume, you will call for the kids to hurry up and brush their teeth with their own homemade wild orange toothpaste and make a mental note to use the immune support rollerball on them before they venture out into the early winter air.

After they leave for school, you'll push the button on your diffuser and the calming scents of lavender and ylang ylang will fill the room you unwind with some yoga for 30 minutes. Then, back in the swing, as you gather a basketful of laundry and...oh no! There sits yesterday's load of towels still in the dryer and not quite dry. You reach for your spray bottle of witch hazel and lemon, spritz some on your wool dryer balls, and add an extra 30 minutes to the cycle to nix any funk that developed overnight. You load up the washing machine and marvel that it only takes a tablespoon of your newly mixed homemade laundry detergent to do what the expensive store brand did—and maybe even a better job! Kitchen cleaning is next on the docket, and you use your homemade dish detergent to battle through the pile of that morning's dishes while getting a burst of awakening aromatherapy from the grapefruit-lemon essential oil blend. Popping open the dishwasher releases a steamy citrus aroma into the kitchen as you unload the shining, streak-free dishes into the cabinets.

When the kids roll in that afternoon, your darling daughter reveals that she somehow managed to get some gum stuck in her hair at recess, but it's nothing that a little lemon oil can't fix. While you get them some healthy snacks, your son sneezes several times in a row and he feels a bit warm to the touch. You reach in your bathroom cabinet for the Cooldown Rollerball Blend (page 86) and then mix up a new rollerball with the intense immunity support provided by the essential oils of oregano, melaleuca, and frankincense. You roll it on the bottoms of their feet, but give some more to your son a few hours later and again before bedtime. That night, after spritzing their pillows with some Sleepy-Time Spray (page 183), you double-check to be sure that they all have a silicone tube of immune support hand cleansing gel in their backpacks and stick a little note in their lunch boxes reminding them to "rub before grub."

The stress of the evening has left you with a glorious headache, so you roll on a tension relief blend to your temples and the back of your neck and debate whether or not to try out your new bath salts. Instead, the hubby offers to give you a foot massage, the perfect opportunity to use the new calming rub you just made. Unfortunately, that idea was short-lived because he complains of pulling a muscle in his back that day, and you end up trying out the Joint and Muscle Soothing Blend (page 91) on his back and then apply a warm washcloth on top to push the oils down in a bit deeper. You rub some lavender on your own feet and add a touch of clary sage as you realize your breasts are beginning to ache, a sure sign that Mother Nature is about to pay a monthly visit. Retiring to bed, you remember to set the timer on your diffuser and drift away into a restful night's sleep, not worried about chemicals, toxins, or any such horrors in your home.

Incorporating essential oils in place of other chemicals and products isn't as daunting a task as it may initially seem. You can make it a family project and begin to replace products one by one in your everyday routine. Your kids will love selecting oils for their own shampoos and body washes, and will begin to learn what oils work for specific needs. You will be empowering your children to develop their own natural routines and surround them with an environment that supports their overall wellness. There are several things that you need to remember when beginning to develop a routine of daily use. Here are ten essentials about essential oils:

1. PROFESSIONAL SUPPORT: No one can substitute a trusted healthcare professional's knowledge and advice when it comes to introducing and utilizing essential oils in your daily routine. In addition, the oils do affect our bodies on a systemic level, so if you have a preexisting health issue, are under a doctor's care for any health issue, or are taking prescription or over-the-counter medication or supplements, be sure to understand how the oils may potentially help, hinder, or interact with this treatment. That said, a lot of essential oil usage has to do with your personal understanding and experience, as well as your intuition as to what is the best option for you.

2. POTENCY: Essential oils are powerful and volatile substances super-concentrated by specific processes. Always keep in mind that less is more when working with essential oils. In a world where more always seems to be better, essential oils need to be delicately utilized and diluted for the best results. Be sure that you understand proper dilution and cross contamination, and remember that a small dose is always the best way to start. One drop of high-quality peppermint essential oil is the same as 28 glasses of peppermint tea!

3. VARIETY: Because many of the essential oils share primary constituents, they are often recommended to achieve the same benefits. But due to the complexity of the other constituents working within each oil and the physical composition of your body, each oil will can cause a different effect for each person, and often, a different effect at different times for the same person. Because of this, I recommend never giving up on a particular oil, but giving it another try. Try out many different oils and oil blends, and don't forget about layering the oils for added benefit. Working the oils into your healthcare and beauty products will give you additional results as well. Finally, apply the oils in different places or try a combination of topical application, aromatherapy, and diffusion to see how the results may differ. It is an individual process for each person, but it will benefit you greatly in the end if you stick to a variety of options.

4. QUALITY IS KEY: High-quality therapeutic pure essential oils must be used to achieve the benefits discussed in this book. Anything else will only introduce inferior quality and results. Watch out for those red flags of adulteration mentioned in Chapter 1. Be sure that you test the oils for quality yourself by doing a simple sniff test or the drop-on-paper test (see page 15). In contrast, an adulterated oil will produce a stain with longevity on the paper. Do your research using the guidelines provided in this book and find a company that you trust. For me, it is a company that not only produces and strictly tests their essential oils, but one that creates partnerships with the farmers, workers, and production companies in the indigenous countries where the products are grown for an overall mutually beneficial relationship.

5. CARE WITH KIDDOS: Children are not tiny adults. We cannot just assume that reducing a recipe will be exactly what our kids need. After discussing essential oil usage with your trusted healthcare professional, you also need to be hyperaware and sensitive to your child's responses and reactions to any new oil, even if it is one that you have used before. Do a patch test whenever you are introducing a new oil. Always dilute when using the oils with kids. Never leave the oils where a child can access them without your permission. I support teaching your children about essential oils and proper application techniques, but this should never be done in an unsupervised capacity. Essential oils affect our moods, our emotions, and our bodies, so know that an emotional release may be triggered by the use of an oil. I recommend keeping a notebook of the oils that you use with your kids and how they respond to them each time. This will help to develop an oil usage routine for them.

6. WATER AND OIL: The rule of thumb to remember is that water and oil repel. They don't get along and will do whatever they can to stay separated. If you want to drive an oil in deeper to an area, a warm or cold wet compress will do an amazing job of getting the oil to that deep spot. But, if you get an essential oil somewhere that causes a reaction or someplace that it doesn't feel comfortable, never try to wash it off! You should add a carrier oil to dilute the oil further and then wipe it off as best as possible.

7. GLASS CONTAINERS: Because of their constituents and super-concentrated nature, essential oils have the potential to eat through certain plastics and materials. Always store your essential oils in glass bottles and use recommended rollerball tops, spray tops, and orifice reducers, which are usually formulated with a specific kind of plastic. When storing your oils, take special care not to leave stray drips on wood, plastic, or any kind of delicate finish. When I first started out, I set a bottle of lavender essential oil on a wooden ledge and later noticed a ring where the bottom of the bottle had been. A stray drop of oil must have dripped down the sides and eaten the white paint away.

8. NO PATENTED ESSENTIAL OILS: Although essential oils have been used for thousands of years in a variety of cultures and continue to be prevalent in many areas of the world, they are rarely utilized in our Western culture. Because they are completely natural, essential oils cannot be patented, making it virtually impossible for pharmaceutical companies to create a profit from them. Mainstream laboratories are more focused on synthetic blends of natural constituents for use in medicines and in the perfume and food industries. Since there very few scientists doing studies on essential oils, most healthcare professionals are hesitant to recommend their usage without clear findings as to their efficacy. We rely on information passed down from very few professionals and many more users for the information that we have today.

9. ESSENTIAL OILS ARE NOT OILY: Because essential oils are derived from volatile compounds in plants, they do not contain the fatty acids that we associate with the word "oil." As a result, they should never feel oily at all, which would be a surefire sign of adulteration. They do blend well with other fatty oils, or carrier oils, that help in the dilution process.

10. BLENDS CREATE SYNERGY: When done correctly, blending essential oils together can create a powerful therapeutic result. The synergy created from blending essential oils with similar therapeutic properties and chemical constituents can provide an amazing benefit to you. Combining the oils together often provides more benefit than the single oils could offer on their own. The few essential oil companies that I trust put painstaking work into the development and testing of new blends each year. The blends that I recommend in this book have been recommended by trusted professionals, and each one has been personally tested. Only you can discover how the blends will work on you as an individual, so approach them with the same caution as you would a single oil.

25 Must-Have Oils

In the following list, I have carefully selected essential oils that I think would make a fantastic starter collection for any family. Pay careful attention to the scientific names, primary constituents, methods of extraction, and countries of sourcing, as this information should be found on the highest quality therapeutic essential oils. Differing information from what I have provided here should be a red flag for adulteration or lower quality essential oil.

1. BASIL—*Ocimum basilicum*

Primary constituents: Linalool

Extraction: Steam distillation of leaves

Country of sourcing: US

Pairs well with: Citrus oils like bergamot, lemon, grapefruit, and lime, as well as clary sage, rosemary, geranium, peppermint, cedarwood, ginger, marjoram, lavender, and wintergreen

Basil's tension-reducing properties, which come from its primary constituent linalool, make it an ideal choice for finding balance in your mind and body. It can reduce anxious feelings while providing a calming focus to your overall well-being. Many people diffuse basil to improve their state of mind and increase their motivation, and meditation with basil helps to restore confidence. It is no wonder that the Italians historically used basil as a symbol of love. A great choice for massage when combined with a carrier oil, basil creates a slight cooling sensation to the skin that helps melt away any pent-up tension and reduce cramping. It is also prized for providing support for the ears when placed on a cotton ball or massaged outside the ear canal. A culinary must-have for foodies, basil provides an amazing addition to your oil collection.

Safety precautions: Pregnant and breastfeeding women should not use basil. Persons with epilepsy should avoid basil as well. Dilute at least 1:1 when using with kids.

Tips for use:

🌿 Use basil with a carrier oil to provide menstrual support during that time of the month.

🌿 Use for post-workout cooldowns. Combine basil and wintergreen with coconut oil and massage over targeted areas for an amazing cooling and tingling sensation that will release tension and open your mind.

❦ Diffuse basil to promote clarity of thought and maintain an open mind. Combine with other complementary oils for an amazing calm.

❦ Ear discomfort? Trying putting a drop of basil on a cotton ball and inserting it overnight in the ear. For an extra kick, add a drop of melaleuca as well. (Essential oils should never be dropped directly into the ear.) You can also massage around the outside of the ear as well.

2. BERGAMOT—*Citrus bergamia*

Primary constituents: Limonene and linalyl acetate

Extraction: Cold pressed from the rinds

Country of sourcing: Italy (Sicily)

Pairs well with: Lavender, patchouli, lime, cypress, eucalyptus, geranium, ylang ylang, and arborvitae

A cross between a lemon and a sour orange, bergamot's distinct aroma not only uplifts your mood, but also offers a dramatic calming effect. When used in massage, bergamot promotes relaxation and helps to alleviate feelings of sadness and anxiety. Many people love to use this oil in their skincare products due to its purifying, cleansing, and soothing properties in addition to its amazing smell. Diffusing bergamot unleashes a spicy citrus scent with a high floral note that steamrolls your negative energy and uplifts your attitude, especially when paired with other calming oils. Another interesting tidbit is that bergamot makes Earl Grey tea; add a drop of bergamot to regular black tea, and voila! Its calming properties also extend to tummy issues, making it a great addition to a rollerball for belly woes, or combined with coconut oil for a calming and uplifting massage.

Safety precaution: Avoid direct sunlight for at least 72 hours after topical application. Bergamot is extremely phototoxic.

Tips for use:

❦ Use bergamot combined with coconut oil for an amazing massage to relax muscle cramping or tension during that time of the month.

❀ Spa sensation! Add bergamot to your body wash or lotions for an uplifting kick in the morning or a calming soothe in the evenings.

❀ Tummy troubles? Try a diluted bergamot massage for soothing a little's belly ache.

❀ Diffuse bergamot with peppermint for a great pick-me-up in the morning, or to help kiddos focus during study time.

❀ Need to create a calming mood for some high-spirited kiddos? Diffuse bergamot with ylang ylang, geranium, or lavender for an ultimate calming combo.

3. CARDAMOM—*Elettaria cardamomum*

Primary constituents: Terpinyl acetate, 1,8-cineole, linalyl acetate, sabinene, and linalool

Extraction: Steam distillation from seeds

Country of sourcing: Guatemala

Pairs well with: Cinnamon, clove, ginger, cedarwood, sandalwood, vetiver, fennel, patchouli, ylang ylang, and citrus oils like bergamot and wild orange

Spicy, fruity, and warm, cardamom is known as the "queen of spices" in the culinary world, where it is an expensive addition to any recipe, especially in India. Similar to ginger, cardamom benefits the digestive system, providing relief from occasional stomach discomfort by slowing down muscle contractions in the intestines. Cardamom also provides powerful support for even the tiniest of respiratory systems, promoting clear breathing and respiratory health. Diffusing cardamom will provide you with mental clarity and openness while calming and soothing your mind and body. It leaves behind a cooling sensation on your skin, but the aroma will help to soothe any areas in need.

Tips for use:

❀ Cozy home! Add a few drops of cardamom to your homemade potpourri or room spray for a warming seasonal scent.

❀ Even for babies, cardamom can be used to ease respiratory distress. Dilute with a carrier and apply to their feet, paying attention to their toes and the bridges of their feet. You can apply it directly to the backs and chests of older kiddos or you can make an amazing chest balm for those winter months.

🌿 Rub diluted cardamom around the belly button to soothe occasional belly issues for any age.

🌿 Clear the mind! Meditate, pray, or read while diffusing cardamom with wild orange or lemongrass for an amazing focus and calm.

4. CEDARWOOD—*Juniperus virginiana*

Primary constituents: Alpha-cedrene, cedrol, and thujospene

Extraction: Steam distillation of the wood

Country of sourcing: US

Pairs well with: Bergamot, eucalyptus, wintergreen, melaleuca, clary sage, rosemary, cypress, and frankincense

Early Egyptians used cedarwood in a variety of ways, from cosmetics to insect repellents to even an embalming agent. Today we use this camphor-rich oil with a woody base note to soothe our minds and bodies. The aroma alone often arouses feelings of vitality and overall wellness, while promoting overall relaxation and easing nervous tension in kids and adults alike. A key grounding oil, the sesquiterpenes provide emotional balance so that you can naturally find your calm. Particularly prized as a natural insect repellent, cedarwood makes a great addition to your gardening routine to protect your plants from hungry predator bugs. The camphor aroma supports respiratory discomfort by opening airways and helping you to breathe deeper. And who doesn't want some healthy skin? Cedarwood promotes a beautiful complexion, so adding it to your beauty products—and your husband's manscaping tools—will keep the both of you glowing and healthy all year round.

Safety precaution: Do not use during pregnancy. Not for children under six years of age.

Tips for use:

🌿 Add some drops of cedarwood to topsoil or mulch and let the aroma ward off unwanted garden pests.

- Add a drop or two of cedarwood to a cotton ball and strategically place around your attic or chests to keep moths and other bugs from feasting on your clothes.

- Preteen males can use a little cedarwood pit pump to keep the stink away. Simply add to some coconut oil or use in a natural deodorant recipe with melaleuca and other essential oils. Your growing boys will love the manly scent!

- Amp up your workout! Athletes in the family will love the addition of cedarwood to their workout routine as it can open up airways and promote vitality. Simply massage a drop or two right onto your chest before the workout.

- Nervous energy? Cedarwood's calming and grounding effect can help to ease nervous tension in unfamiliar surroundings. Simply add a drop to your palms and inhale, or sniff right from the bottle. This is a great relief for introverts who may begin to come undone in new environments (especially during those middle school years!). Diffusing it can also promote feelings of confidence and self-esteem.

- Add a drop or two to any moisturizer to clarify skin tone and promote relaxation.

- Adding a bit of cedarwood to your hair care products, along with thyme, rosemary, and/or lavender, can help to stimulate hair follicles. Also create the Rich Coconut Oil Hair Mask on page 132 with those essential oils and some coconut oil. Massage in and let it work for three minutes before washing out.

5. CLARY SAGE—*Salvia sclarea*

Primary constituents: Linalyl acetate and linalool

Extraction: steam distillation of flower

Countries of sourcing: US and northern Mediterranean

Pairs well with: Roman chamomile, geranium, frankincense, cypress, sandalwood, lavender, peppermint, rosemary, and citrus oils like lemon, lime, and wild orange

This biennial or perennial herb has been used since the Middle Ages for its calming benefits for the skin and deeply relaxing effects on the body. It is prized by midwives for use during childbirth, but pregnant women should avoid contact with clary sage until they are ready to meet their baby. Of utmost importance is the use of clary sage to support a woman's body during her special time of the month. It can soothe and calm many women's issues while helping the body find a hormonal balance. Add it to your skincare regimen or use it for a massage with a carrier oil. No matter how you use it, this oil is a must-have for all of the females in your family!

Safety precautions: Take caution during pregnancy. Use only during childbirth, as it can cause uterine contractions. Not for use with children.

Tips for use:

- Apply clary sage to your pulse points for relief during your most stressful times...and especially once each month!

- Diffuse away the sass! Before you snap at the kiddos, try diffusing clary sage with grapefruit and lime as a great mood-boosting pick-me-up during the sassiest of days.

- Try homemade herbal hairspray. Clary sage with geranium, peppermint, rosemary, lavender, and sugar water make an easy solution for unmanageable hair. Not only will it make your coif gorgeous, but it will also provide an amazing aromatherapeutic solution all day long.

- Apply some clary sage to your pillow before bedtime and let the calming aroma relax you away into a restful night's sleep.

- If that time of moth has you wishing you could go back to bed and curl into a ball, try a bit of clary sage massaged into your abdomen or back for relief from menstrual pains.

- Every mama needs a relaxing bath, so swirl some Epsom salt with lavender, Roman chamomile, and clary sage into your bathwater and let the stress melt away.

6. CLOVE—*Eugenia caryophyllata*

Primary constituents: Eugenol

Extraction: Steam distillations of buds

Country of sourcing: Madagascar

Pairs well with: Basil, rosemary, rose, cinnamon, nutmeg, peppermint, lavender, geranium, and citrus oils like lemon, grapefruit, and wild orange

Harvested from the buds of the evergreen tree, clove comes from the Latin *clovus*, meaning "nail," for its appearance. Not just used to spice up your hams, clove provides a warm and spicy aroma for any time of year. Historically, it has been renowned as a breath freshener by the Chinese and then as a pest deterrent in Europe during the plague. Added to your oral hygiene products, clove can add an amazing punch to your breath and the natural warming/numbing effect can soothe irritated gums. The men in your life will appreciate the addition of clove to their personal care products as it will not only provide a musky, long-lasting aroma, but will also keep bugs away naturally. It is also prized for its immune-supporting properties and powerful antioxidants. And don't forget its amazing autumn aroma—diffusing clove can make your home smell like the season!

Safety precautions: Clove is a hot oil and has a natural numbing effect. It should always be diluted when used, at least 1:1 for adults and 1:4 for children over the age of six. Do not use for kids under the age of six. Caution should also be taken during pregnancy. Cloves can irritate sensitive skin.

Tips for use:

- Garden protection! Work some clove oil into your topsoil or mulch for an all-natural bug repellent.
- Add clove to your mouthwash for a soothing and numbing effect. You can also dab diluted clove on the gums to soothe sore gums.
- Toothpaste boost! Add drops of clove to your Whitening/ Remineralizing Toothpaste (page 139) to enhance your oral health. Kids may not enjoy the taste, but it is great for adults who are bored with mint.
- Add clove to your homemade potpourri for a seasonal kick, or diffuse it with some cinnamon and wild orange to spice up your home.

🌿 Spicy scrub! Add clove, ginger, cinnamon, and wild orange to white or brown sugar and coconut oil. Not only will this support your body's immune system, but it will also exfoliate your body and provide an amazing tingling sensation for the roughest of days.

7. EUCALYPTUS—*Eucalyptus radiata*

Primary constituents: Eucalyptol and alpha-terpineol

Extraction: Steam distillation of leaves

Country of sourcing: Australia

Pairs well with: Citrus oils like lemon and wild orange, and peppermint or other minty oils

Often over 50 feet high, sky-ticking eucalyptus trees are known as "gum trees" to natives of Australia. The camphorous, airy aroma of eucalyptus promotes feelings of clear breathing and open airways, while its amazing skin purification properties make it a popular addition to many beauty products. It also has a place in supporting oral hygiene and makes a powerful breath freshener that has the added benefit of respiratory support. Eucalyptus adds an amazing addition to any massage, as it supports the skin and reduces tension in the body. Many people prefer its aroma in their hard surface cleaners and use it as a natural air freshener. When combined in vinegar and water with other essential oils like peppermint, wild orange, or lemon, eucalyptus serves as a powerfully aromatic cleanser for even the stinkiest, gunkiest areas of your home.

Safety precaution: Take caution with kids under the age of six years old due to the potential of high menthol content to slow breathing.

Tips for use:

🌿 Get a natural glow. Add a few drops to your daily moisturizer for a soothing and purifying result.

🌿 Winter doldrums? Diffuse eucalyptus with some citrus oil to revitalize your mind and spirit during those dull winter months.

🌿 Itchy, dry scalp? Eucalyptus mixed with coconut oil can create a tingly scalp massage that will help to alleviate dry skin.

- Along with melaleuca, eucalyptus can help to both prevent and get rid of nasty outbreaks of lice. As soon as you hear that four-letter word at your kid's school, add a bit of either oil to your palm and smooth it in their hair to repel those little nasties!

- Purify the air in your home either by diffusing eucalyptus, adding it to a room freshener spray, or adding a drop or two to your vacuum filter before sucking up the dirt.

- Eucalyptus also makes an amazing spot remover for dirt, grease, or gunk. Keep some by your laundry station for those everyday what-the-heck-is-that? moments.

- Combined with lavender, cypress, frankincense, and melaleuca in some coconut oil and beeswax, eucalyptus can provide a powerful salve for a variety of needs while relaxing away stress.

8. FENNEL—*Foeniculum vulgare*

Primary constituents: E-anethole, fenchol, and alpha-pinene

Extraction: Steam distillation from seeds

Country of sourcing: Egypt

Pairs well with: Cinnamon, sandalwood, geranium, lavender, and citrus oils like lime

The ancient Romans ate fennel in preparation for battle, as they believed it would fill them with strength and longevity. The ancient Egyptians used it to combat snakebites. This versatile essential oil has a strong black licorice smell laced with sweet honey tones and is prized for supporting healthy digestion. It may promote a healthy respiratory function when applied to the chest and can also support the respiratory tract. Many people use fennel for promoting healthy circulation, liver function, and circulation throughout the body. The licorice flavor also seems to help cut cravings and minimize hunger for those trying to keep a healthy lifestyle. Many say it can even keep you away from processed sugar and sweets.

Safety precautions: Use with caution during pregnancy or if being treated for epilepsy. Dilute at least 1:1 when using with kids. Repeated contact with the skin may cause desensitization.

Tips for use:

🌿 After a huge meal or a stressful event, massage diluted fennel into the belly or circle around the belly button to relieve any belly stress and support healthy digestion.

🌿 Feeling sluggish or bloated? Fennel can help to support your metabolism.

🌿 Losing focus? Diffusing fennel with geranium or rosemary can help to boost your productivity and increase your sense of focus. It will energize you and help you to find your confidence.

🌿 Dip a toothpick in diluted fennel essential oil and then keep it in your mouth to minimize hunger and cravings.

🌿 For flavoring, be sure to dip a toothpick in fennel essential oil and then swirl it into your creation, otherwise it will overpower the entire dish.

🌿 Nursing mama? Use fennel to support milk production! Apply a diluted rollerball of fennel right to the ladies, or, if the scent is too much, apply to the bottoms of your feet.

9. FRANKINCENSE—*Boswellia carterii/frereana/sacra*

Primary constituents: Alpha-pinene, limonene, and alpha-thujene (beta-pinene)

Extraction: steam distilled from the resin

Countries of sourcing: Somalia, Ethiopia, Oman, and Yemen

Pairs well with: Most oils, including citrus oils like lemon, lime, wild orange, and grapefruit, as well as sandalwood, cypress, geranium, rose, ylang ylang, and clary sage

Known as the "king of essential oils," frankincense has been prized since biblical times for its deep, spicy earth notes and incense overtones. The name comes from the old French *franc encens*, meaning quality incense, and is sometimes called olibanum. When it comes to rejuvenating your skin and reducing the appearance of imperfections, nothing supports your complexion more than this amazing essential oil. Not only does it support healthy cellular function throughout the body, but it also promotes a healthy inflammatory response while contributing to an overall feeling of wellness. The warm spicy aroma has also been used for supporting respiratory health, especially when blended synergistically with other essential oils. Its applications for emotional balance and spiritual wellness are endless, as it has been used for centuries to focus energy while improving meditation and awareness. It is no wonder that frankincense is many people's desert-island oil—the one oil that they cannot be without.

Tips for use:

- Warm up the holidays. What better scent to waft around during your holiday celebrations? Diffuse it with a bit of wild orange for a sweet spice that your family will love.

- Stretch marks? Scars? Try dabbing on some frankincense for a few weeks and watch as the imperfections slowly fade away. Perfect for even the most accident-prone kiddos!

- For a healthy glow, add some frankincense to your daily moisturizer or cleanser to rejuvenate your complexion.

- Massage some frankincense with coconut oil into your kiddos' hands and feet after hardcore snow play to create a soothing, warming feeling.

- Frankincense diffused or applied topically is a great way to focus your intentions for the day or direct your kids' study efforts to the task at hand. It is also a great addition to morning or evening prayer routines or meditation/yoga/workout routines.

- Nasty chest gunk? Layer lime, then cardamom, then frankincense on the chest, back, and feet of littles to alleviate stress and tension from constant coughing and promote respiratory health. You can swap the cardamom with peppermint or eucalyptus for older kiddos. To intensify the effect, apply a warm compress on top to drive the oils in deeper and create a steamy aromatherapy benefit.

- Tension? A self-care foot massage with frankincense can help to dispel negative feelings and stress while returning your positive attitude. Every mama needs a little TLC!

10. GERANIUM—*Pelargonium graveolens*

Primary constituents: Citronellol, citronellyl formate, and geraniol

Extraction: Whole plant steam distillation

Country of sourcing: Mauritius

Pairs well with: Lavender, rosemary, basil, cedarwood, and citrus oils like bergamot, wild orange, lemon, lime, and grapefruit

Mostly prized for its beauty as a flower, geranium has been used for centuries as a fix for flawed complexions and even a breath freshener. Its aroma is similar to that of the rose due to its primary constituent, geraniol, and it is often used as a substitute for rose in many perfumes and products. Many beauty products use geranium for its soothing effects on skin blemishes and issues. Diffusing it will not only help you to release stress, but will also promote feelings of peace and hope. Women have also prized geranium for its calming properties during labor. Used as an aphrodisiac, geranium can be an amazing addition to a massage oil. It can be used to promote relaxation and leave your skin feeling silky smooth in the process.

Tips for use:

❀ Add a drop or two of geranium to your favorite moisturizer for a double-effect of calming your skin and providing you with an amazing aroma all day long.

❀ Geranium, when added to your Homemade Natural Deodorant (page 130), will give you a feminine scent and leave you with silky-smooth pits in the process.

❀ Geranium is an all-natural bug repellent, so add it to your DIY bug sprays for an extra floral kick.

❀ Get healthy hair! Add a drop or two of geranium to your shampoo or conditioner and be amazed at the transformation of your mane.

❀ Diffuse geranium with citrus or herbal blends for an amazing calming scent to help calm the entire family.

❀ Diffuse or apply geranium to calm your body and mind during moments of tension during labor.

❧ Mix geranium with witch hazel and dab on hemorrhoids with a cotton ball to soothe the irritation.

11. GRAPEFRUIT—*Citrus X paradisi*

Primary constituents: D-limonene

Extraction: Cold pressed from rinds

Country of sourcing: US

Pairs well with: Frankincense, ylang ylang, geranium, lavender, peppermint, rosemary, and bergamot

Named for its clustered growing structure, grapefruit essential oil hits top notes with citrus and floral scents that uplift and motivate. When inhaled or diffused, grapefruit has a clarifying effect on the mind and provides an overall balance to the body. It is also prized for its amazing cleansing ability due to its high limonene content, which is known for its ability to dissolve oils. From hand cleaners to surface sprays to skincare products, grapefruit packs a punch of purifying power. Many people use grapefruit in their beauty products, as it promotes clear and healthy skin while also supporting a healthy metabolism. Just inhaling grapefruit can help to curb cravings and increase your motivation to stay on track. It is also popular for diffusing, especially when combined with other uplifting or focusing oils. Women love grapefruit for its ability to aid in areas that could use some smoothing and tightening. No matter how you choose to use it, the balance that grapefruit provides to the body and mind make it an essential component for every family.

Safety precaution: Grapefruit is a phototoxic oil. Avoid direct sunlight for at least 12 hours after application.

Tips for use:

❧ Late night? Diffuse grapefruit with peppermint to kick your body into action in the morning and provide focus to your day.

❧ For teens, grapefruit is a great choice for spot treatments of blemishes, or you can make a toner with witch hazel, grapefruit, melaleuca, and lavender to calm and soothe the skin.

❧ A grapefruit massage can help to melt away feelings of tension and uplift your attitude.

- Add grapefruit to the DIY Rejuvenating Pink Salt Scrub, Lavender and Honey Body Wash, or Homemade Citrus Body Butter recipes found in Chapter 6 for an amazing skin smoothing and soothing experience.

- Diffuse or apply grapefruit to help kids focus on the task at hand as they study for a test.

- It's great for diet support! Inhaling grapefruit can help you to stay focused during the day or before workouts, and may make any cravings a thought of the past.

12. HELICHRYSUM—*Helichrysum italicum*

Primary constituents: Neryl acetate, alphapinene, and gamma-curcumene

Extraction: steam distillation of flower

Country of sourcing: France (Corsica)

Pairs well with: Melaleuca, myrrh, frankincense, geranium, clary sage, lavender, and citrus oils

Packed full of powerful esters, the sweet honey-like scent of helichrysum renews the mind and body like no other essential oil. Known as the "everlasting flower" or "immortal flower," it was prized by the ancient Greeks for its herbal remedies and ability to rejuvenate the complexion. As a result, you can find it in many antiaging products as it promotes a healthy, youthful, and glowing complexion. Not only does it provide a soothing sensation to the skin, but it also can fade the appearance of stretch marks and scars while promoting the regeneration of healthy skin cells. For emotional balance, helichrysum is used to unblock resistance and calm feelings of anger, while uplifting and uncluttering the subconscious mind. Many people refer to helichrysum as first aid in a bottle.

Tips for use:

- Support a healthy complexion by combining helichrysum with jojoba oil and targeting those age spots. This also works well with acne scars or spots, dark pigmented skin, and stretch marks.

- Make your own Soothing Salve (page 131) for razor burns by adding helichrysum to the recipe. Dab on areas of concern after shaving.

- Nothing is more stressful for a teen than a surge of acne on their body. Helichrysum can provide complexion support when applied topically on target areas. Dab the oil on your finger and use as an on-the-go everyday spot treatment.

- Low energy? Use helichrysum for an energizing massage with a carrier oil that will provide full-body support and promote vitality.

- Diluted helichrysum on a cotton ball can provide soothing relief from the terrible side effects of hemorrhoids either during pregnancy, after pregnancy, or at any time of life.

- Aromatherapy! Add a drop or two of helichrysum to any of your DIY cleaners for an amazing boost of herbaceous aroma.

13. LAVENDER—*Lavandula angustifolia*

Primary constituents: Linalool and linalyl acetate

Extraction: Steam distillation of flower

Country of sourcing: France

Pairs well with: Most oils, including citrus oils like bergamot and lime, and herbaceous oils like marjoram and basil

In medieval times, lavender was prized for its applications when dealing with love, though the debate between aphrodisiac and chastity kept people busy. Ancient Romans and Egyptians utilized this tension-busting aroma for everything from relaxing baths to cooking and perfuming their world. Today, lavender is prized for its light floral scent, filled with calming esters that can soothe both the mind and body. Lavender essential oil doesn't have the hardcore floral scent that you may be used to in synthetically scented products, so you may be surprised at the powdery fragrance that whisks you away into dreamland. When in doubt, lavender will probably be the answer due to its wide range of applications. From promoting emotional balance and returning feelings of peace to gently supporting the natural glow of your skin, lavender is a must-have in your collection of essential oils.

Safety precaution: Some people claim that lavender use can cause breast growth in prepubescent boys. Studies conflict on this finding, but be aware in case you notice this side effect.

Tips for use:

❦ Try the Restful Sleep Spray (page 94) on bedclothes, pillows, and stuffed animals before bed to create a serene environment for a restful night's sleep.

❦ Diffuse a few drops or massage a few drops into your pulse points for a quick, tension-relieving fix to your day. If you have the time, a lavender bath soak will melt away built-up tension and help to restore a positive and peaceful mood.

❦ Boost your beauty products, including body wash, cuticle cream, lip balm, and others. Lavender helps to support dry skin and reduces the appearance of skin imperfections.

❦ Dealing with razor burn? Lavender and coconut oil will help keep away that sandpapery itch.

❦ Try adding a few drops of lavender to a potpourri or make your own in the spring and summer with seasonal flowers and herbs. You can even add a drop or two in the cardboard tube of a roll of toilet paper, and experience a fresh scent every time you roll!

❦ Add lavender and water to a spray bottle and spray down a yoga mat to help ward of the sweaty funk. It will also produce a relaxing aroma while you bend and stretch. For an extra bonus, massage a drop of lavender on the back of your neck before beginning your routine.

❦ If you find yourself a little lobstery after too much time in the sun, a spritz or rub of lavender with frankincense and peppermint will help to support your skin's health and provide a calming, cooling effect wherever it is applied.

❦ You will be amazed at how quickly lavender can ease and support your skin's recovery from even the nastiest of bug bites. Your kids will thank you again and again for a rollerball with lavender and fractionated coconut oil for easy application. It's a must-have for bug season or if you frequent the outdoors.

❦ Lavender is so mild that it can be used in even the tenderest of situations. Diffusing lavender or having a lavender massage can ease you through the contractions of childbirth and even help to promote a restful night's sleep in those uncomfortable last few months of pregnancy. Once your little one has passed the three-month mark, lavender can support him or her through many uncomfortable growing pains, from teething to bellyaches and gas.

- ✤ Add a drop of lavender to your mascara when it gets gunky for a revitalized formula that will not only go on smoother, but also come off easier.

14. LEMON—*Citrus limon*

Primary constituents: Limonene, beta-pinenes, and gamma-terpinene

Extraction: Cold-pressed from the rinds

Country of sourcing: Italy (Sicily)

Pairs well with: Lavender, peppermint, eucalyptus, fennel, geranium, grapefruit, bergamot, lime, Douglas fir, wintergreen, cinnamon, and wild orange

For centuries, lemons have been painstakingly cultivated and carefully and lovingly grown by trusted farmers who have passed down their knowledge from generation to generation. Lemon essential oil should have a clean and bright, citrus-fresh scent that invigorates and enlivens the mind and body. Known as a powerful cleansing agent, its antioxidant properties not only ward off free radicals and toxins in your home, but also purify the air and surfaces as you use it as a nontoxic cleaner. Diffusing it provides an uplifting and energizing mood booster that will refresh your mind and ward off negativity, especially when paired with the essential oils listed above.

Safety precautions: Lemon oil is phototoxic and must be used with care when exposed to direct sunlight. Be sure to dilute it before use and avoid direct sun exposure for at least 12 hours after application on your skin.

Tips for use:

- ✤ Spring got you down? Combine with equal parts peppermint and lavender to support seasonal respiratory discomfort.
- ✤ Mix with water in a glass spray bottle for an easy shake-and-spritz hard surface cleaner and odor eliminator. Works great to get rid of oily fingerprints on stainless steel appliances!

- Add to olive oil or coconut oil and apply to scratched or scuffed wood furniture.

- Gum in hair? Stickers on glass? Sap in clothes? Use as an all-purpose anti-sticking agent.

- Add to everyday detergent or soap as an instant degreaser or hard water combatant.

- Carefully apply to your hair for DIY highlights in the summer.

- Put a few drops on a cotton ball and stick in areas with undesirable aromas (gym bags, shoes, trash cans).

- Forgot your towels in the dryer? Add a few drops of lemon oil to a wet washcloth and throw in to revive the load.

15. LEMONGRASS—*Cymbopogon flexuosus*

Primary constituents: Geranial and neral

Extraction: Steam distillation from leaves

Country of sourcing: India

Pairs well with: Basil, cedarwood, coriander, geranium, lavender, melaleuca, spearmint, and cardamom

Though its name may confuse you, lemongrass contains no actual citrus and comes from a grass-like plant. Its strong lemony-citrus fragrance adds zing to many Asian dishes while promoting digestive health. The pungent aroma also heightens awareness and promotes a positive outlook on life. It has found a home in many beauty care products for its purification of the skin and toning properties. Many massage therapists have also harnessed the power of lemongrass to soothe the body after exertion and leave their clients with a refreshed feeling. When used with your DIY cleaners, lemongrass provides an amazing aroma while cleansing surfaces. It makes a great addition to your collection, as it can also be used to balance out the aroma of blends, especially when using them topically in the summer when you want to avoid phototoxic lemon or other citrus oils.

Safety precaution: Dilute at least 1:1 if using when pregnant or with children.

Tips for use:

- Lemongrass is a natural bug repellent and cuts the harsh smell of peppermint when used as a bug spray.

- Lemongrass is great for a post-workout massage when combined with a carrier. Work it into areas of heavy exertion for soothing relief and a refreshed feeling.

- Happy belly! Combine lemongrass with peppermint or cardamom to provide digestive relief for occasional stomach upset.

- Diffuse lemongrass to kick nervousness to the curb and to energize your mind and body. It will both heighten your awareness and promote a positive outlook to get you through the toughest times, especially when combined with other grounding and uplifting oils.

16. LIME—*Citrus aurantifolia*

Primary constituents: Limonene, beta-pinene, and gamma-terpinene

Extraction: Cold pressed from rinds

Country of sourcing: Brazil

Pairs well with: Clary sage, lavender, rosemary, ylang ylang, and other citrus oils

The citrusy-tart smell of lime often sends our thoughts to the tropics, especially when combined with unrefined coconut oil. Not only is lime a great scent to diffuse for energizing your mind and body, but it also uplifts the mood and provides balance overall, especially when combined with other essential oils. Like its other citrus counterparts, lime's primary constituent is limonene, making it a powerful addition to your cleaning products. Its purifying capabilities for the air, combined with its uplifting scent, make it a favorite for use in and out of the home. It is also great for providing respiratory support during those winter months when coughs sometimes get out of control. You can find lime in many facial and body cleansers and products for its amazing scent and it's ability to cut through oil, making pale skin brighter.

Safety precautions: Avoid direct sun exposure for at least 12 hours after applying lime topically as it is phototoxic. Use at least a 1:1 dilution ration with children.

Tips for use:

- Mood boost! Diffuse lime with peppermint or other citrus oils for a quick pick-me-up.

- Lime breaks down the gunk and stick in many kid-favorite products. Add a bit of lime to gum stuck in hair or shoes. Massage it in, then wipe away. Also great for sticker gunk left behind on windows or other undesirable areas.

- Apply a drop of lime to grease stains to work out in the laundry.

- Chest gunk? Apply the Respiratory Support Rub Blend (page 100) to the chest and back. This is especially helpful at night to promote sleep.

- Create a sugar scrub with an amazing beach-like aroma by using unrefined coconut oil, white sugar, and lime essential oil that will be a favorite no matter what season.

17. MARJORAM—*Origanum majorana*

Primary constituents: Terpinen-4-ol, sabinene hydrate, Y-terpinene and gamma-terpinene

Extraction: Steam distillation of leaves

Country of sourcing: Hungary

Pairs well with: Bergamot, lavender, rosemary, cedarwood, Roman chamomile, cypress, eucalyptus, and melaleuca

Known as "wintersweet" or "joy of mountains" to the Greek and Romans, marjoram symbolized joy and happiness for many ancients. It is also interestingly called "goose herb" by the Germans because they use it to roast geese in their culinary specialties. The calming properties of marjoram make it a popular choice for promoting sleep and peace, whether applied topically or diffused. It may also promote healthy cardiovascular health and provide support for the immune system. Providing emotional balance enables marjoram to have a positive effect on the nervous system as well. Overall, lessening feelings of stress and reducing discomfort without side effects are the main reasons people love having marjoram in their essential oil collection.

Safety precautions: Use with caution during pregnancy. Dilute at least 1:1 when using with kids.

Tips for use:

- 🌿 Fussy kiddo? Apply diluted marjoram to the bottoms of your kiddo's feet to promote calm. Add some lavender or Roman chamomile for some extra peace.
- 🌿 Massage marjoram into your targeted muscle areas both before and after your workouts.
- 🌿 Massage marjoram with clary sage into your abdomen to relax tense muscles during your favorite time of the month.
- 🌿 For those bumps on the head, shins, and any other place, try adding marjoram to the Bump Relief Blend (page 89) and apply every few hours as needed.

18. MELALEUCA—*Melaleuca alternifolia*

Primary constituents: Terpinen-4-ol and gamma-terpinene

Extraction: Steam distillation of leaves

Country of sourcing: Australia

Pairs well with: Citrus oils like lemon, lime, and wild orange, as well as cypress, eucalyptus, lavender, rosemary, and thyme

Most commonly known as tea tree oil, melaleuca is prized for its cleansing and purifying constituents that are not only used in cleaning products but also in a whole array of beauty and personal care products. Native to Australia, crushed melaleuca in a variety of different compounds has been used by the Aborigines for years to heal cuts, wounds, and skin infections. Melaleuca promotes a healthy immune function and can be used in a pinch with any skin irritation or concern, especially in combination with lavender or other essential oils. As a hard surface cleaner, this herbaceous essential oil can protect your home from environmental threats while also purifying and freshening the air. Diluted, it is also a staple oil to have in your cabinet for use with every member of your family.

Safety precautions: Melaleuca is poisonous if swallowed in large quantities, so keep it away from children. May irritate sensitive skin. Dilute when using if bothered by the cooling effect that it creates.

Tips for use:

🌿 Teens and moms alike will love the ease of melaleuca for spot treatments when dealing with skin imperfections from acne.

🌿 Mani/pedi at home! Dilute with some coconut oil and paint on a bit of melaleuca to promote healthy, fresh cuticles and nails before your mani/pedis.

🌿 Create your own low-cost facial toner by mixing 10 drops of melaleuca in two ounces of witch hazel.

🌿 Hair bugs? Lice outbreaks at school can be a parent's and a kid's worst nightmare. Be on the offensive by spritzing your kiddo's mane with melaleuca and water and keeping any long hair tightly pulled back. It can also be used as a spritz around the house in case of an outbreak. Add a drop or two to the family's hair care products for added prevention.

🌿 Add melaleuca and lemon to vinegar and water for an everywhere cleaner and deodorizing spray. Great for preventing mold on shower doors as well.

🌿 Add melaleuca to Homemade Natural Deodorant (page 130) for purification and odor prevention.

🌿 DIY diaper cream! Add melaleuca and lavender to coconut oil for an amazing Soothing Baby Skin Balm (page 105) for your babies. It is also an amazing cream for girls of all ages who need a little help down under.

🌿 Melaleuca is a must-have in your first aid kit as it helps to purify the skin and cleanse the area around the wound. Do not apply directly to the wound. Add some lavender and frankincense for extra support.

19. OREGANO—*Origanum vulgare*

Primary constituents: Carvacrol and thymol

Extraction: Steam distillation of leaves

Country of sourcing: Turkey

Pairs well with: Lavender, rosemary, bergamot, Roman chamomile, cypress, cedarwood, melaleuca, and eucalyptus

Used for centuries for its potent and powerful results, oregano provides a powerful ally for supporting your immune system. This herbaceous and camphorous sharp scent goes a long way however you choose to use it. Oregano also supports healthy digestion for occasional issues. Known as an amazing cleaning agent, many people add this oil to their DIY cleaning recipes for an extra kick. When added to blends of oils, it acts as an enhancer and equalizer and provides a punch of antioxidants. Oregano's powerful aroma can also support respiratory function, soothing the lungs and helping to break up the junk. Because of its intense warming effect and aroma, many people avoid using oregano, but you cannot go wrong when including it in your immune support blends as it strengthens your vital centers and enhances feelings of security. It is one of the oils that should always be diluted due to its strong effect and potential to irritate the skin, so be sure to do a patch test before using it in anything.

Safety precautions: Take caution when using due to potential burns on the skin. Oregano must be heavily diluted by everyone who uses it. Use at least a 1:3 oil to carrier ratio with adults and do not use on children under the age of six. Take caution when using with kiddos and apply to their feet before using on other areas of their bodies; you do not want them getting oregano in their eyes or mouths! Pregnant women should use caution as well. Avoid getting it near mucous membranes and eyes, and if you feel any irritation, immediately dilute with more oil and add lavender to soothe your skin. I also would not apply after a hot shower when your pores would be open.

Tips for use:

- 🌿 Kick up cleaning! Add a drop or two of oregano to your Multiple-Purpose Cleaning Spray (page 115) for extra protection.
- 🌿 Combine oregano with frankincense, rosemary, and melaleuca, and dilute with a carrier oil. Apply daily for an awesome immune-supporting blend. Great for those winter months!

❦ For a powerful sinus-clearing experience, add a drop each of oregano, peppermint, lime, and eucalyptus to very warm water. Be sure to cover your nose and mouth with a washcloth before leaning over the steamer to avoid getting the steam in your eyes.

20. PEPPERMINT—*Mentha piperita*

Primary constituents: Menthol, menthone, and 1,8-cineole

Extraction: Whole plant steam distillation

Countries of sourcing: US (Washington), Europe, and Asia

Pairs well with: Lemon and lavender for seasonal support, as well as oregano, marjoram, cypress, eucalyptus, rosemary, geranium, grapefruit, and juniper berry

A plant hybrid of water-mint and spearmint, peppermint continues to keep us on our toes due to its distinguishing high menthol content. Prized for its use in oral hygiene products, peppermint has found a steady home in toothpastes, mouthwashes, and chewing gums, though most of these products use a synthetic peppermint with its distinctly sweet candy-cane-like smell. High-quality peppermint essential oil provides unparalleled support for healthy respiratory function and clear breathing, though it is not recommended for use in children under six years of age. When applied topically, its cooling sensation can help the body cool down when overheated. It is also known for alleviating occasional stomach discomfort due to its ability to relax the bowels and reduce bloating and gas. This minty and herbaceous aroma can enliven the senses and bring focus back to your day while energizing you to keep going. Even in moments of muscle tension, peppermint's tingly cooling effect can soothe and calm aching muscles. And it is a must-have for every family due to its ability to repel most insects and rodents!

Safety precautions: Caution is advised for pregnant or nursing women, and those being treated for high blood pressure or epilepsy. Also use caution if you are taking other medication for digestive health. If you are taking iron as a supplement, do not use peppermint within a three-hour period of taking your iron. Not recommended for kids under the age of six years due to the high menthol content's potential to slow breathing.

Tips for use:

- After a long day of standing or a rough night of little sleep, use the aroma of peppermint to pique your senses and leave you feeling energized. For an extra punch, diffuse with uplifting grapefruit and grounding sandalwood to balance your day.

- To give your family a get-up-and-go boost in the early morning hours or keep you alert during long drives, try diffusing peppermint with wild orange. This is also a great blend for focus during studying.

- If you skimped out on the sunscreen and can still feel the heat coming off of your burning skin, try a spray of peppermint, lavender, and frankincense for a cooling, relaxing solution.

- Add peppermint to distilled water in a small glass spritzer bottle for a cooldown spray at the beach. It will also help you to maintain healthy-looking skin. Recommended for older kids and adults only.

- Peppermint with a bit of lemongrass will keep the nastiest of bugs away from your family and your house. Spritz weekly in dark corners and along baseboards and doorframes to keep the spiders and ants from making themselves at home. You can even spray your window screens and around the outside of your home as well.

- Place peppermint oil on cotton balls and stick under cabinets and in areas where rodents may find entry during those winter months or in the summer when they are looking for a snack.

- Diluted lavender, lemon, and peppermint can keep the woes of seasonal distress from transforming you into a snotty, swollen mess. Simply dab behind your ears and diffuse in your house to support your entire family during this time of itch.

- Great for scalp massage. Add a couple drops of peppermint to your shampoo or conditioner to support a healthy scalp and to give you an added tingle when washing your hair.

- A peppermint foot massage not only helps to reduce any odor but will provide a tingly relaxation to any aching feet.

- Stuffed up? Try putting a drop or two of peppermint on your shower floor. The steam will lift up the menthol and help to alleviate your respiratory discomfort.

21. ROMAN CHAMOMILE—*Anthemis nobilis*

Primary constituents: 4-methylamyl angelate, isobutyl angelate, and isoamyl tiglate

Extraction: Steam distilled from flower

Country of sourcing: US

Pairs well with: Lavender, ylang ylang, geranium, patchouli, clary sage, and citrus oils like bergamot, grapefruit, lemon, and lime

One of the safest and most calming essential oils available, Roman chamomile was used by the ancient Romans to give them courage and clear minds during times of war. Today, we often use chamomile in our herbal teas for that same type of calm. Amp up that power by utilizing Roman chamomile essential oil in everything from your beauty products to massage oil. Not only does it help to support healthy sleep, but it also can ease discomfort for a variety of childhood issues. Even for those times of temper tantrums and lack of focus, Roman chamomile can be applied topically or diffused to help calm and bring focus back to kiddos. This is a must-have oil if you value peace and emotional stability in your home.

Tips for use:

❀ Can't sleep? Apply Roman chamomile to the bottoms and/or tops of your feet to promote a restful night's sleep. For a more powerful kick, layer it with some lavender and diffuse in the room, too!

❀ Ease the crankiness and irritability in your home by diffusing Roman chamomile. It will provide a soothing effect for the entire house with its calming floral tones and create a peaceful environment for everyone.

❀ For kiddos or parents in a funk, applying Roman chamomile to pulse points can help to soothe the soul and clear the mind of conflict.

❀ Roman chamomile makes a great addition to any facial mask or moisturizer and can even be a welcome addition to shampoo and conditioner. Use it daily on your skin for soothing.

✤ Wear Roman chamomile as an amazing perfume to keep you comforted and calm through even the tensest of situations. This works great for those rough middle school and high school years as well.

22. ROSEMARY—*Rosmarinus officinalis*

Primary constituents: 1,8-Cineole, alpha-pinene, and camphor

Extraction: Steam distillation of flower and leaves

Country of sourcing: Morocco

Pairs well with: Frankincense, lavender, clary sage, cedarwood, basil, thyme, lemongrass, geranium, peppermint, and cardamom

Sacred in many ancient civilizations, rosemary was used for protection from the plague and for fumigating evil spirits. Today, it finds a home in many culinary masterpieces as well. Rosemary can promote healthy digestion and internal organ function when applied in times of need. Many people like to include it in their hair care products, as it may promote hair growth. Its energizing scent can be diffused to reduce nervous tension and soothe away any anxious feelings. Occasional fatigue can also be thwarted either by diffusing it with complementary oils or by applying it topically. Many people use it to stimulate the mind and memory, open the conscious mind, and maintain concentration. This makes it the perfect solution for kiddos who need to focus on the task at hand or if there is a big test and they need to study. A word of caution though: this oil is not a good choice for workaholics or high-strung people, as it is very stimulating and will only drive them harder!

Safety precautions: Avoid rosemary when pregnant. Dilute to at least 1:1 with kids. Persons being treated for epilepsy or high blood pressure should also avoid rosemary.

Tips for use:

✤ A quick circle of rosemary around the belly button will help to calm occasional discomfort due to gas.

✤ Diffuse rosemary with wild orange to focus the mind on the task at hand. Great for kiddos who would benefit from some calming focus.

- Thinning hair? Add rosemary to hair care products or as a spot treatment on particular areas to stimulate follicles and support hair growth.

- Combine rosemary, lemon, and bergamot in the Natural DIY Conditioner (page 133).

- Rosemary can be a solution to promote oral hygiene when combined with a mouth rinse or toothpaste if you don't mind the herbaceous scent and taste.

23. WILD ORANGE—*Citrus sinensis*

Primary constituents: Limonene

Extraction: Cold pressed from the rinds

Country of sourcing: Dominican Republic

Pairs well with: Peppermint, frankincense, geranium, lavender, cinnamon, clove, ginger, sandalwood, vetiver, and black pepper

Though wild orange may seem to be a simple scent, its fresh citrus aroma is packed full of monoterpenes that stimulate the mind and body, as well as support a healthy immune system. Like other citrus oils, wild orange makes a great addition to any of your homemade cleaners as it purifies the air and surfaces while cutting down grease and gunk. It also uplifts the mind and body when diffused and enhances most other essential oil blends. It has also been prized in its ability to support digestive health while also providing immune support when threats are high. Many people also find it to be a delightful addition to recipes when a little tart citrus kick is needed.

Safety precaution: Wild orange is phototoxic and direct UV rays should be avoided for at least 12 hours following topical application.

Tips for use:

- Combine wild orange with peppermint and frankincense for a great focusing diffuser blend that will boost your mood and keep you motivated.

- Adding some wild orange to a bit of vinegar and water will create a degreasing, de-gunking powerhouse spray that can be used in everything from grimy toilets to sticky countertops.
- Never underestimate the enlivening aroma of wild orange, as it makes a great air freshener for even the funkiest funks.
- Have a kiddo that is full of anxiety over a test, a performance, or a dental exam? Have him or her inhale the aroma of wild orange for an uplifting and calming experience.
- Cranky baby? Wild orange can also ease upset in babies when it is diluted and massaged into their feet or on their stomach to alleviate occasional discomfort.

24. WINTERGREEN—*Gaultheria fragrantissima/procumbens*

Primary constituents: Methyl salicylate

Extraction: Steam distillation from leaves

Countries of sourcing: Nepal (*fragrantissima*) and China (*procumbens*)

Pairs well with: Oregano, thyme, basil, bergamot, cypress, geranium, lavender, lemongrass, marjoram, and ylang ylang

Harvested from the muddy foothills of Nepal, wintergreen requires such specific growing requirements that it is one of the lowest essential oil yielding plants known. As a result, it is often adulterated, so only buy from a trusted company that performs quality checks and uses strict standards. Wintergreen has been used as a flavoring for a variety of oral health products as well as in root beer in the food industry. It is also prized for its ability to ease muscle and joint pain. When applied topically, its warming effect will help to relax tension, as it may naturally cause a numbing sensation and then feel cool to the skin. Be sure to always dilute wintergreen when using it in topical creams or massage blends.

Safety precautions: Avoid use during pregnancy. Highly poisonous if ingested, the essential oil bottle should come with a childproof cap. Individuals being treated for epilepsy should also avoid contact with this oil.

Tips for use:

* Create a soothing muscle rub for the athletes or elderly members of your family by combining wintergreen with some coconut oil.

* Place a drop or two of wintergreen on a cotton ball and place in areas where stink reigns.

* Swirl some Epsom salt into warm bathwater and add wintergreen and lavender for a soothing bath experience.

25. YLANG YLANG—*Cananga odorata*

Primary constituents: Germacrene and caryophyllene

Extraction: Steam distillation of the flower

Country of sourcing: Madagascar

Pairs well with: Geranium, marjoram, sandalwood, vetiver, and citrus oils like bergamot, grapefruit, and lemon

Steam-distilled from unique star-shaped flowers, ylang ylang has been used in many religious and wedding ceremonies, providing an aphrodisiac quality with its intoxicating aroma that also promotes mental and emotional balance. It can lift your mood while also promoting calm throughout the mind and body. Ylang ylang can promote a positive outlook on life when diffused and alleviate any lingering feelings of anger or stress. Many people add it to hair and skincare products for its amazing aroma as well as its nourishing and protecting properties. For stress relief, you can't go wrong with ylang ylang, especially when blended with other essential oils like lavender, bergamot, or vetiver.

Tips for use:

* Mix a few drops of ylang ylang in an Epsom salt bath for a relaxing evening soak.

* To release bacteria and dirt from your skin, try a steam facial with ylang ylang. Combine very warm water with a few drops of oil and tent your head over the bowl. Its sweet scent will relax your mind and body while purifying your skin.

* Make your own special scent by combining ylang ylang with complementary scents for a unique aroma. Remember the final step

to testing perfume is to apply to your skin, as each person's body chemistry works differently with the essential oil aromas.

❧ Itchy scalp? In the heat of summer, massage a few drops of ylang ylang into the scalp to calm and soothe.

❧ Add ylang ylang to coconut oil to create a deep hair conditioner.

❧ Ylang ylang layered with lavender and vetiver can promote a powerfully peaceful sleep for all ages. Start with ylang ylang on its own and then add lavender. If that still isn't enough to get you or your kiddos some Z's, add a bit of vetiver to the mix.

CHAPTER

4

SMART MOM RECIPES FOR EVERYDAY EMERGENCIES

Being a smart mom means being prepared for bumps, owies, tantrums, and hot mess moments with natural solutions that are safe for the entire family, including you. Tears, sticky hands, and meltdowns are mixed in with laughter, family celebrations, and cuddles. Prepare for the struggles and triumphs of the day with just a handful of essential oils, a carrier oil, and some rollerball bottles. This chapter is filled with effective smart mom recipes, ranging from diffuser blends to bath soaks and rollerball bottle solutions that are easy to make and use at a moment's notice. You will find the rollerball bottle recipes to be ideal for everyday emergencies, and easy to store in your purse.

The recipes and blends included in this chapter are specially formulated for kids one to five years old (two percent dilution), six to 11 years old (five percent dilution), and 12 to 17 years old (10 percent dilution). I recommend starting with a low dilution rate for all three groups, and you can always add more essential oil to the blend to make it more potent. Remember to always do a patch test on your kids when using new oils to check for any skin sensitivity. You can always try several different areas of application, but remember that the bottoms of the feet are an excellent location for younger kids.

In some recipes, I substitute spearmint for peppermint in the blends to avoid the high menthol content. Spearmint is a safer alternative for children under 12 years old. For adults, peppermint is an effective choice. As I mentioned in Chapter 1, one drop of peppermint essential oil is the equivalent to 28 glasses of peppermint tea, which makes it very potent and effective.

I do not recommend using essential oils on babies three months and younger. You will find essential oil blends specifically for babies at the end of this chapter. Always be careful when applying oils on babies and children and perform a skin patch on yourself and your baby before applying them.

When implementing these solutions for yourself and your family, feel confident that you are providing effective and safe natural solutions that are incredibly convenient to implement. You do not need to know every single constituent for each essential oil in order to effectively use it on yourself and your family. Simply remember that essential oils are some of the greatest plant resources for supporting the human body on a physical and emotional level.

In case you are hungry to learn more about the essential oils used in these recipes, be sure to check out the 25 Must-Have Oils on page 48.

Rollerball Blends

Note: For each 10-milliliter rollerball bottle, you will need approximately 2 teaspoons of carrier oil.

TEMPORARY DIGESTIVE UPSET RELIEF BLEND

Peppermint, spearmint, and ginger are effective at easing temporary nausea. Ginger and fennel relieve stomach discomfort. This blend is ideal in a rollerball bottle for easy use, especially during travel, or after eating foods that don't agree with you. The blend provides fast-acting relief. It is also beneficial for promoting a healthy gastrointestinal tract.

YIELD: 10-milliliter rollerball bottle

FOR 1 TO 5 YEARS OLD (2% DILUTION)
2 drops ginger essential oil
2 drops fennel essential oil
Carrier oil of choice

FOR 6 TO 11 YEARS OLD (5% DILUTION)
4 drops ginger essential oil
4 drops fennel essential oil
2 drops spearmint essential oil
Carrier oil of choice

FOR 12 TO 17 YEARS OLD (10% DILUTION)
8 drops ginger essential oil
8 drops fennel essential oil
4 drops spearmint or peppermint essential oil
Carrier oil of choice

DIRECTIONS: Add essential oils to rollerball bottle and top off blend with a carrier oil of choice. Apply this blend directly over the small and large intestines to ease temporary digestive upset.

MOTION SICKNESS BLEND

Peppermint, spearmint, and ginger are effective at reducing temporary nausea, especially on long car rides or boat trips.

YIELD: 10-milliliter rollerball bottle

FOR 1 TO 5 YEARS OLD (2% DILUTION)
3 drops spearmint essential oil
1 drop ginger essential oil
Carrier oil of choice

FOR 6 TO 11 YEARS OLD (5% DILUTION)
7 drops spearmint essential oil
3 drops ginger essential oil
Carrier oil of choice

FOR 12 TO 17 YEARS OLD (10% DILUTION)
15 drops peppermint or spearmint essential oil
5 drops ginger essential oil
Carrier oil of choice

DIRECTIONS: Add essential oils to rollerball bottle and top off blend with a carrier oil of choice. Inhale ginger and spearmint/peppermint every 15 to 30 minutes. Apply to mastoid area behind the ears once an hour until discomfort passes.

TEMPORARY STOMACH INDIGESTION BLEND

The combination of peppermint/spearmint and fennel is effective at reducing temporary indigestion after spicy meals.

YIELD: 10-milliliter rollerball bottle

FOR 1 TO 5 YEARS OLD (2% DILUTION)
2 drops spearmint essential oil
2 drops fennel essential oil
Carrier oil of choice

FOR 6 TO 11 YEARS OLD (5% DILUTION)

5 drops spearmint essential oil

5 drops fennel essential oil

Carrier oil of choice

FOR 12 TO 17 YEARS OLD (10% DILUTION)

10 drops peppermint or spearmint

10 drops fennel essential oil

Carrier oil of choice

DIRECTIONS: Add essential oils to rollerball bottle and top off blend with a carrier oil of choice. Apply to the stomach and near the sternum/esophageal area every hour until discomfort subsides.

SOOTHING BLEND FOR IRRITATED SKIN AND MINOR BURNS

Lavender is effective at calming skin and removing heat from the skin's surface. Helichrysum further supports lavender for promoting healthy skin.

YIELD: 10-milliliter rollerball bottle

FOR 1 TO 5 YEARS OLD (2% DILUTION)

2 drops lavender essential oil

2 drops helichrysum essential oil

Carrier oil of choice

FOR 6 TO 11 YEARS OLD (5% DILUTION)

5 drops lavender essential oil

5 drops helichrysum essential oil

Carrier oil of choice

FOR 12 TO 17 YEARS OLD (10% DILUTION)

10 drops lavender essential oil

10 drop helichrysum essential oil

Carrier oil of choice

DIRECTIONS: Add essential oils to rollerball bottle and top off blend with a carrier oil of choice. Apply to very minor skin irritations every 30 minutes to rapidly soothe skin.

Note: Only apply to minor skin irritations. Seek medical assistance for serious skin issues.

SEASONAL RESPIRATORY DISCOMFORT BLEND

Equal parts of lemon, lavender, and peppermint/spearmint essential oils are known for their ability to promote clear breathing and support a healthy immune response when combined. Used by both veteran and novice essential oil users, this well-known blend is frequently used for its head and respiratory health benefits.

YIELD: 10-milliliter rollerball bottle

FOR 1 TO 5 YEARS OLD (2% DILUTION)
2 drops lavender essential oil
1 drop lemon essential oil
1 drop spearmint essential oil
Carrier oil of choice

FOR 6 TO 11 YEARS OLD (5% DILUTION)
5 drops lavender essential oil
3 drops lemon essential oil
2 drops spearmint essential oil
Carrier oil of choice

FOR 12 TO 17 YEARS OLD (10% DILUTION)
7 drops lavender essential oil
7 drops lemon essential oil
6 drops peppermint essential oil
Carrier oil of choice

DIRECTIONS: Add essential oils to rollerball bottle and top off blend with a carrier oil of choice. Roll the blend behind the ears and on the back of your neck; also try over your feet, and up and down the back.

SOOTHING BUG BITE BLEND

YIELD: 10-milliliter rollerball bottle

FOR 1 TO 5 YEARS OLD (5% DILUTION)
5 drops lavender essential oil
5 drops melaleuca (tea tree) essential oil
Carrier oil of choice

FOR 6 TO 11 YEARS OLD (25% DILUTION)
25 drops lavender essential oil
25 drops melaleuca (tea tree) essential oil
Carrier oil of choice

FOR 12 TO 17 YEARS OLD (50% DILUTION)
50 drops lavender essential oil
50 drops melaleuca (tea tree) essential oil
Carrier oil of choice

DIRECTIONS: Add essential oils to rollerball bottle and top off blend with a carrier oil of choice. Dab the blend over bug bites, or roll on areas of concern.

These are very high concentrations of essential oils, but the blend is targeted to a very specific area and you need very little over the bite. Dab on the bite every 2 hours to soothe the area. Also, you do not need to use a rollerball bottle to make this blend. You can store the blend in an empty bottle and apply 1 drop as needed.

COOLDOWN ROLLERBALL BLEND

Lavender is effective at supporting the immune system while assisting peppermint or spearmint in providing a cooling sensation.

YIELD: 10-milliliter rollerball bottle

FOR 1 TO 5 YEARS OLD (2% DILUTION)
3 drops lavender essential oil
1 drop spearmint essential oil
Carrier oil of choice

FOR 6 TO 11 YEARS OLD (5% DILUTION)

7 drops lavender essential oil

3 drops spearmint essential oil

Carrier oil of choice

FOR 12 TO 17 YEARS OLD (10% DILUTION)

15 drops lavender essential oil

5 drops peppermint essential oil

Carrier oil of choice

DIRECTIONS: Add essential oils to rollerball bottle and top off blend with a carrier oil of choice. Apply to bottoms of feet and spine to promote cooling when overheated. Apply every 1 to 2 hours.

EAR SOOTHE ROLLERBALL BLEND

YIELD: 10-milliliter rollerball bottle

FOR 1 TO 5 YEARS OLD (2% DILUTION)

2 drops lavender essential oil

1 drop basil essential oil

1 drop melaleuca essential oil

Carrier oil of choice

FOR 6 TO 11 YEARS OLD (5% DILUTION)

6 drops lavender essential oil

2 drops basil essential oil

2 drops melaleuca essential oil

Carrier oil of choice

FOR 12 TO 17 YEARS OLD (10% DILUTION)

12 drops lavender essential oil

4 drops basil essential oil

4 drops melaleuca essential oil

Carrier oil of choice

DIRECTIONS: Add essential oils to rollerball bottle and top off with carrier oil. Apply 2 to 3 drops from bottle to a cotton ball and gentle apply a small amount behind the ear, on the mastoid, and around the front of the ear. Keep it there for 10 minutes, being careful to not place directly in ear canal, then remove from ear. Continue to apply to ear every hour until it feels better.

OWIE BLEND

Lavender calms irritated skin. Melaleuca and frankincense promote healthy skin. This blend can also be made into a spray with distilled water or carrier oil in a 2-ounce spray bottle.

YIELD: 10-milliliter rollerball bottle

FOR 1 TO 5 YEARS OLD (2% DILUTION)
2 drops lavender essential oil
1 drop melaleuca essential oil
1 drop frankincense essential oil
Carrier oil of choice

FOR 6 TO 11 YEARS OLD (5% DILUTION)
4 drops lavender essential oil
3 drops melaleuca essential oil
3 drops frankincense essential oil
Carrier oil of choice

FOR 12 TO 17 YEARS OLD (10% DILUTION)
8 drops lavender essential oil
6 drops melaleuca essential oil
6 drops frankincense essential oil
Carrier oil of choice

DIRECTIONS: Add essential oils to rollerball bottle and top off with carrier oil of your choice. Dab onto a clean finger and apply to area of concern.

ENERGIZER BOOST BLEND

Citrus essential oils contain monoterpenes, which have energizing and revitalizing benefits, making them ideal for instantly boosting energy. Citrus essential oils are also powerful for promoting a healthy immune system.

YIELD: 10-milliliter rollerball bottle

FOR 1 TO 5 YEARS OLD (2% DILUTION)
2 drops wild orange essential oil

2 drops spearmint essential oil

Carrier oil of choice

FOR 6 TO 11 YEARS OLD (5% DILUTION)
5 drops wild orange or grapefruit essential oil

5 drops spearmint essential oil

Carrier oil of choice

FOR 12 TO 17 YEARS OLD (10% DILUTION)
10 drops wild orange or grapefruit essential oil

10 drops peppermint or spearmint essential oil

Carrier oil of choice

DIRECTIONS: Add essential oils to rollerball bottle and top off with carrier oil of your choice. For a quick energizing boost, apply blend behind the ears or to back of neck throughout the day.

BUMP RELIEF BLEND

YIELD: 10-milliliter rollerball bottle

FOR 1 TO 5 YEARS OLD (2% DILUTION)
1 drop geranium essential oil

1 drop frankincense essential oil

1 drop cypress essential oil

1 drop helichrysum essential oil

Carrier oil of choice

FOR 6 TO 11 YEARS OLD (5% DILUTION)
4 drops geranium essential oil

3 drops frankincense essential oil

3 drops cypress essential oil

1 drop helichrysum essential oil

Carrier oil of choice

FOR 12 TO 17 YEARS OLD (10% DILUTION)
6 drops geranium essential oil

5 drops frankincense essential oil

5 drops cypress essential oil

3 drops helichrysum essential oil

Carrier oil of choice

DIRECTIONS: Add essential oils to rollerball bottle and top off with carrier oil of your choice. Apply 2 to 3 drops to area of concern to relieve temporarily raised and irritated skin.

NECK AND HEAD TENSION RELIEVER

YIELD: 10-milliliter rollerball bottle

FOR 1 TO 5 YEARS OLD (2% DILUTION)
2 drops frankincense essential oil

2 drops lavender essential oil

Carrier oil of choice

FOR 6 TO 11 YEARS OLD (5% DILUTION)
5 drops frankincense essential oil

5 drops lavender essential oil

Carrier oil of choice

FOR 12 TO 17 YEARS OLD (10% DILUTION)
10 drops frankincense essential oil

10 drops lavender essential oil

Carrier oil of choice

DIRECTIONS: Add essential oils to rollerball bottle and top off with carrier oil of your choice. Roll the blend over your neck, back, temples, and top of forehead and rub the blend into skin. Avoid the eyes by applying to the very top of forehead and dabbing on finger to apply to temples.

Note: For adults, I recommend adding peppermint essential oil to the blend for cooling relief.

JOINT AND MUSCLE SOOTHING BLEND

Lavender, frankincense, and basil added to spearmint provides relief to muscles and joints. Increase the effectiveness of this recipe by applying a warm compress after applying the essential oil blend. This blend is ideal for post-sport activities, workouts, and during growth spurts.

YIELD: 10-milliliter rollerball bottle

FOR 1 TO 5 YEARS OLD (2% DILUTION)
1 drop lavender essential oil
1 drop frankincense essential oil
1 drop spearmint essential oil
1 drop marjoram essential oil
Carrier oil of choice

FOR 6 TO 11 YEARS OLD (5% DILUTION)
3 drops lavender essential oil
3 drops frankincense essential oil
2 drops spearmint essential oil
2 drops marjoram essential oil
Carrier oil of choice

FOR 12 TO 17 YEARS OLD (10% DILUTION)
6 drops lavender essential oil
6 drops frankincense essential oil
4 drops spearmint essential oil
4 drops marjoram essential oil
Carrier oil of choice

DIRECTIONS: Add essential oils to rollerball bottle and top off with carrier oil of your choice. Apply soothing blend to tired muscles and joints to relieve tension.

STRESS RELIEF BLEND

You can also diffuse this blend to relieve stress, or diffuse before bed to promote a good night's sleep. Frankincense, lavender, and wild orange elicit a calming aroma for moments of stress, and this blend can be used throughout the day to provide calming support and ease tense feelings. This blend is great as a rollerball blend for mamas when applied to the wrist at a 10 percent dilution.

YIELD: 10-milliliter rollerball bottle

FOR 1 TO 5 YEARS OLD (2% DILUTION)
2 drops lavender essential oil

1 drop frankincense essential oil

1 drop wild orange essential oil

Carrier oil of choice

FOR 6 TO 11 YEARS OLD (5% DILUTION)
4 drops lavender essential oil

3 drops frankincense essential oil

3 drops wild orange essential oil

Carrier oil of choice

FOR 12 TO 17 YEARS OLD (10% DILUTION)
8 drops lavender essential oil

6 drops frankincense essential oil

6 drops wild orange essential oil

Carrier oil of choice

DIRECTIONS: Add essential oils to rollerball bottle and top off with carrier oil of your choice. Apply blend to bottom of feet, back of neck, or spine for reducing stress.

IMMUNE SUPPORT BLEND

YIELD: 10-milliliter rollerball bottle

FOR 1 TO 5 YEARS OLD (2% DILUTION)
2 drops lemon essential oil

1 drop melaleuca essential oil

1 drop clove essential oil

Carrier oil of choice

FOR 6 TO 11 YEARS OLD (5% DILUTION)

3 drops lemon essential oil

3 drops melaleuca essential oil

2 drops eucalyptus essential oil

2 drops clove essential oil

Carrier oil of choice

FOR 12 TO 17 YEARS OLD (10% DILUTION)

6 drops lemon essential oil

6 drops melaleuca essential oil

4 drops eucalyptus essential oil

4 drops clove essential oil

Carrier oil of choice

DIRECTIONS: Add essential oils to rollerball bottle and top off with carrier oil of your choice. Apply to bottoms of feet to prevent environmental threats. You can also use this blend in the diffuser to purify the air, or make a spray out of the essential oils to clean doorknobs and other items that are touched throughout the day.

Sprays

Sprays are not typically broken down into age groups. I created sprays that will work for all ages. However, you will find that the Soothing Throat Spray includes age groups because the spray is applied directly to the throat and the concentration works best when adjusted according age.

BUG OFF SPRAY

Designed to be used for clothes and air, hair and shoes, this blend is great for camping, hikes, and travel. Take it on trips for effective, nontoxic bug protection. Use caution using peppermint with kids under the age of 6. You can replace the peppermint with cedarwood if using with children under the age of 6.

YIELD: 2-ounce glass spray bottle

10 drops peppermint or cedarwood essential oil

5 drops lemongrass essential oil

¾ cup distilled water

DIRECTIONS: Add essential oils and distilled water to spray bottle. Shake to mix blend completely. Spray blend on clothes, shoes, ankles, and in hair to avoid pesky bugs. Also great around the house to keep the bugs out. Take care to avoid the eyes.

RESTFUL SLEEP SPRAY

The Restful Sleep Spray is designed to be sprayed on pillows, not people. Lavender and vetiver are a powerful combination for a restful sleep. Other oils to incorporate include cedarwood, clary sage, and Roman chamomile. Witch hazel evaporates more quickly than water and can be substituted.

YIELD: 2-ounce glass spray bottle

1½ ounces distilled water or witch hazel

10 drops lavender essential oil

5 drops vetiver essential oil

DIRECTIONS: Add water or witch hazel to spray bottle. Add the essential oils, shake, and spritz. Spray on pillows, comforters, and in the air before bed for a restful sleep.

SOOTHING THROAT SPRAY

Peppermint and ginger will provide rapid scratchy throat relief. Lemon essential oil is a powerful immune supporter. Lavender helps to soothe.

YIELD: 4-ounce glass spray bottle

FOR 1 TO 5 YEARS OLD

¾ cup distilled water

5 drops lemon essential oil

1 drop lavender essential oil

1 drop ginger essential oil

FOR 6 TO 11 YEARS OLD

¾ cup distilled water

15 drops lemon essential oil

3 drops lavender essential oil

3 drops ginger essential oil

FOR 12 TO 17 YEARS OLD

¾ cup distilled water

30 drops lemon essential oil

6 drops peppermint essential oil

6 drops ginger essential oil

DIRECTIONS: Add water to spray bottle. Add essential oils and blend by shaking bottle. Shake well before spraying on the back of the neck. Apply every 30 minutes, or as needed. Store up to 3 months.

Epsom Salt Bath Soaks

Due to the amount of water you will be using, the percentages of EO would be significantly less than 1 percent.

IMMUNE-BOOSTING SOAK

Lavender calms tension in muscles. Lavender, lemon, and melaleuca are effective at promoting a healthy immune system. Take 1 bath per day when warding off illness.

YIELD: 1 application

FOR 1 TO 5 YEARS OLD

1 drop lavender

1 drop melaleuca

1 drop lemon

¼ cup Epsom salt

FOR 6 TO 11 YEARS OLD

3 drops lavender

3 drops melaleuca

1 drop lemon

¼ cup Epsom salt

FOR 12 TO 17 YEARS OLD

6 drops lavender essential oil

6 drops melaleuca essential oil

3 drops lemon essential oil

¼ cup Epsom salt

DIRECTIONS: Combine essential oils into a glass bowl to make a blend. Run a warm bath. Combine Epsom salt and essential oil blend and add to bath. Stir with hand and soak in tub for 20 minutes.

RELAXING MUSCLE BATH

Lavender and Roman chamomile help to relax muscles and quiet the mind. Marjoram eases tight muscle tension.

YIELD: 1 application

FOR 1 TO 5 YEARS OLD

2 drops lavender essential oil

1 drop Roman chamomile essential oil

1 drop marjoram essential oil

¼ cup Epsom salt

FOR 6 TO 11 YEARS OLD

3 drops lavender essential oil

2 drops Roman chamomile essential oil

1 drop marjoram essential oil

¼ cup Epsom salt

FOR 12 TO 17 YEARS OLD

6 drops lavender essential oil

5 drops Roman chamomile essential oil

3 drops marjoram essential oil

¼ cup Epsom salt

DIRECTIONS: Combine essential oils into a glass bowl to make a blend. Run a warm bath. Blend Epsom salt into essential oil and add to bath. Stir with hand and soak in tub for 20 minutes.

Diffuser Blends

GET FOCUSED DIFFUSER BLEND

I recommend mixing this blend in an empty amber bottle ahead of time and keeping it by your kitchen diffuser. This blend is great if your kids are having trouble focusing on homework, or maybe when the entire family is working on a project together. This amazing concentration blend can be used on kids and adults alike.

YIELD: 1 application

1 drop spearmint essential oil

2 drops wild orange essential oil

1 to 2 drops of frankincense essential oil

DIRECTIONS: Add essential oil drops to your favorite diffuser and diffuse for 30 minutes to assist with focus and concentration.

MENTAL ALERTNESS DIFFUSER BLEND

Rosemary and grapefruit essential oils are effective at increasing motivation and concentration. Peppermint and spearmint constituents provide rapid alertness when feeling tired or low in energy.

YIELD: 1 application

2 drops rosemary essential oil

2 drops spearmint or peppermint essential oil

1 drop grapefruit essential oil

DIRECTIONS: In a diffuser, apply essential oil drops and diffuse for 30 minutes to one hour to promote mental stimulation. Or, apply 1 drop of each on a cloth napkin and inhale 3 deep breaths as needed.

OPEN AIRWAYS DIFFUSER BLEND

This blend is ideal during bedtime to open up airways and promote a restful night's sleep. For children 12 years and older, also try using peppermint and eucalyptus.

YIELD: 1 application

2 drops cardamom essential oil

2 drops cypress essential oil

1 drop lime essential oil

DIRECTIONS: Add essential oils to a diffuser and diffuse 30 minutes to one hour to open respiratory airways and assist in clear breathing pathways. Or, apply one drop of each to a cloth and take 3 to 5 breaths to clear airways.

Rubs and Gels

CALMING LAVENDER RUB

My two favorite ways to use lavender with kids are topically and aromatically. You can add lavender to raw coconut oil for an essential oil rub after bath time or before bed. Try massaging their feet with it or using it in place of lotion. Lavender can also be combined with other essential oils like bergamot or Roman chamomile.

YIELD: 4-ounce jar

FOR ALL AGES

½ cup raw coconut oil

1 cup hot water

15 drops lavender essential oil

DIRECTIONS: Spoon the coconut oil into a glass jar with a lid (like a Mason jar) and carefully set it in the hot water. Gently stir as the coconut oil melts. Once the oil is completely melted, add the essential oil and stir. Place the glass jar in the refrigerator for an hour until it sets, then keep at room temperature. To use, scoop out and rub in your hands; the oil will melt in your hands from the heat of your body.

Note: Don't wash your hands if you apply the rub to your children! Smart moms and dads can use some calming power, too, so rub it into your hands or on your face at night to promote relaxation and soothe your skin!

IMMUNE SUPPORT HAND CLEANSING GEL

This recipe makes a great gift for the teachers in your lives. Along with this Immune Support Hand Cleansing Gel, never underestimate the power of gifting a diffuser and a bottle of wild orange to your child's classroom! Keeping your immune system in tip-top shape is the first step to keeping your family healthy and safe.

YIELD: 1 reusable 2-ounce silicon tube

FOR AGES 2 AND UP
¼ cup aloe vera gel
½ teaspoon vegetable glycerin
1 tablespoon witch hazel
15 drops melaleuca or wild orange

DIRECTIONS: Combine the ingredients in the tube. Shake until well-blended. Squirt a small amount on your hands and rub together to use.

OVERHEATED COOL COMPRESS

Roman chamomile and lavender in equal qualities make an effective cooling agent. Melaleuca is effective for supporting the immune system.

YIELD: 1 application

FOR AGES 2 AND UP
2 drops lavender
2 drops melaleuca
1 drop roman chamomile
4 cups of lukewarm water

DIRECTIONS: Combine the essential oils in a small bowl and add them to a large bowl containing the lukewarm water. Stir the water to completely mix the essential oils. Use a clean washcloth and make a compress by soaking the washcloth in the solution. Apply compress to the forehead, spine, feet, and torso. Continue applying compresses for 20 minutes. Apply 2 to 4 times a day until the body is cooled down.

RESPIRATORY SUPPORT RUB BLEND

This rub is intended to open up airways by expanding the chest and supporting healthy lung function. This blend is calming and relaxing and can promote restful sleep.

YIELD: 24 applications

FOR 1 TO 5 YEARS OLD (2% DILUTION)

6 teaspoons coconut oil

6 drops lavender essential oil

3 drops cardamom essential oil

2 drops cypress essential oil

1 drop lime essential oil

FOR 6 TO 11 YEARS OLD (5% DILUTION)

6 teaspoons coconut oil

14 drops lavender essential oil

8 drops cardamom essential oil

6 drops cypress essential oil

2 drops lime essential oil

FOR 12 TO 17 YEARS OLD (10% DILUTION)

6 teaspoons coconut oil

28 drops lavender essential oil

16 drops cardamom or eucalyptus essential oil

12 drops cypress essential oil

4 drops lime essential oil

DIRECTIONS: Add the coconut oil along with lavender, cardamom, cypress, and lime essential oils and shake very well to blend the rub. Use your fingers to apply a small amount to the back and neck and massage it into the skin. Repeat the treatment three to four times a day and before bedtime. Store in a dark amber jar in a cool place.

IMMEDIATE SKIN RELIEF SALVE

This blend can also serve as a massage blend to support the immune system. Apply to the spine and bottom of feet.

YIELD: 2-ounce jar

FOR 1 TO 5 YEARS OLD (2% DILUTION)
11 drops lavender essential oil

8 drops helichrysum or frankincense essential oil

6 drops Roman chamomile essential oil

1 drop spearmint essential oil

¼ cup cold-pressed refined coconut oil

FOR 6 TO 11 YEARS OLD (5% DILUTION)
24 drops lavender essential oil

18 drops helichrysum or frankincense essential oil

16 drops Roman chamomile essential oil

3 drops spearmint essential oil

¼ cup cold-pressed refined coconut oil

FOR 12 TO 17 YEARS OLD (10% DILUTION)
48 drop lavender essential oil

36 drops helichrysum or frankincense essential oil

26 drops Roman chamomile essential oil

10 drops peppermint essential oil

¼ cup cold-pressed refined coconut oil

DIRECTIONS: Melt the coconut oil in a double boiler or hot water bath. In a glass jar, add all the essential oils to the coconut oil and gently swirl the jar for the blend to completely mix. Let harden at room temperature or pop in the fridge for quick hardening. Scoop a teaspoon of the mixture out of the jar and rub between your hands to melt the oil, and then apply to areas of concern.

Baby Support

BABY RESPIRATORY BLEND

YIELD: 10-milliliter rollerball bottle

FOR 3 MONTHS TO 2 YEARS OLD
1 drop cardamom essential oil
1 drop frankincense essential oil
1 drop wild orange essential oil
Fractionated coconut oil

DIRECTIONS: Place the essential oil in a 10-milliliter rollerball bottle and then fill to the top with the coconut oil. Roll the blend over bottoms of feet for respiratory support.

PEACEFUL SLEEP

YIELD: 10-milliliter rollerball bottle

FOR 3 MONTHS TO 2 YEARS OLD
2 drops lavender essential oil
1 drop frankincense essential oil
Fractionated coconut oil

DIRECTIONS: Place the essential oil in the rollerball bottle and then fill to the top with the coconut oil. Roll the blend over bottoms of feet to promote a restful and calming sleep.

TEETHING RELIEF

YIELD: 10-milliliter rollerball bottle

FOR 3 MONTHS TO 2 YEARS OLD
1 drop lavender essential oil
1 drop frankincense essential oil
Fractionated coconut oil

DIRECTIONS: Place the essential oil in a rollerball bottle and then fill to the top with the coconut oil. Dab a small amount onto a clean finger and apply along jawline.

BABY DIGESTIVE SUPPORT

YIELD: 10-milliliter rollerball bottle

FOR 3 MONTHS TO 2 YEARS OLD
1 drop cardamom essential oil
1 drop lavender essential oil
1 drop fennel essential oil
Fractionated coconut oil

DIRECTIONS: Place the essential oil in a rollerball bottle and then fill to the top with the coconut oil. Dab a small amount onto a clean finger and apply around belly button or to bottoms of feet.

CRADLE CAP BLEND

YIELD: 1 application

FOR 3 MONTHS TO 2 YEARS OLD
1 drop melaleuca essential oil
1 drop geranium essential oil
2 tablespoons fractionated coconut oil or almond oil

DIRECTIONS: In a small bowl, dilute the essential oils in the carrier oil and massage into your child's scalp, concentrating on the worst areas of cradle cap. Allow the oil to soak in for a couple of minutes to help loosen the scales. Use a baby comb to lightly lift the scales out of the hair.

FRETFUL BABY BLEND

Babies get fretful, and this blend will help them feel calm and relaxed. Give the baby a gentle massage after applying to the feet or spine to promote calm.

YIELD: 10-milliliter rollerball bottle

FOR 3 MONTHS TO 2 YEARS OLD
1 drop geranium essential oil
1 drop Roman chamomile essential oil
Fractionated coconut oil or almond oil

DIRECTIONS: Place the essential oils in the rollerball bottle and then fill to the top with your carrier oil of choice. Apply to bottom of feet and to the spine.

BABY COOLDOWN BLEND

This can be applied every 15 to 30 minutes until the baby cools down.

YIELD: 10-milliliter rollerball bottle

FOR 6 MONTHS TO 2 YEARS OLD
1 drop spearmint essential oil
1 drop lavender essential oil
Fractionated coconut oil

DIRECTIONS: Place the essential oils in a rollerball bottle and then fill to the top with the coconut oil. Apply to bottom of feet and/or to the spine.

PATOOTIE BALM

YIELD: 8-ounce jar

FOR 3 MONTHS TO 2 YEARS OLD
12 drops lavender essential oil
6 drops melaleuca essential oil
1 cup raw organic coconut oil

DIRECTIONS: Melt the coconut oil in a glass jar in a water bath. Add in the oils and stir. Solidify in the refrigerator. Rub in after diaper changes to promote healthy skin.

SOOTHING BABY SKIN BALM

YIELD: 8-ounce jar

FOR 3 MONTHS TO 2 YEARS OLD
8 drops lavender essential oil
6 drops Roman chamomile essential oil
1 cup raw organic coconut oil

DIRECTIONS: Melt the coconut oil in a glass jar in a water bath. Add in the oils and stir. Solidify in the refrigerator. Gently massage on areas of need.

CHAPTER

❧5❧

GREEN RECIPES FOR THE HOME

Is your cleaning routine really as clean as you think it is? Have you ever stopped to look at the ingredients list on any of your everyday household cleaners? I'm not talking about the hardcore, spring cleaning, grout-busting stuff—just the normal things you use for countertops and toilets.

That laundry list of unpronounceable chemicals and endocrine disruptors should concern you when it comes to your family's health. The toxic chemicals found in most cleaning products on the market today may cause both short- and long-term health issues, especially when we consider children. Because their bodies are still developing, certain chemicals may interfere with numerous systems in their bodies, especially their endocrine system. Surely you keep your cleaning supplies locked up, but have you thought about exposure from breathing the fumes or simply touching a countertop?

Respiratory rates in younger children are higher than those of adults, so they absorb more air contaminants than we do. And if that isn't scary enough, how about this alarming statistic: The US Environmental Protection Agency says that the air inside our homes is typically 200 to 500 percent more polluted than the air outside! Why? Toxic household cleaning products persist in our household environment in our carpets, countertops, and floors.

Rest assured, you can make over your entire cleaning routine in a few hours and with just a handful of staple green cleaning products, most of which you probably already have in your house. Not only are these ingredients highly effective, but they are also very cost effective. Even better, you only need a few products to tackle the entire spectrum of dirt and grime in your house, rather than bottle after bottle of specific retail products.

Essential oils are some of the best-smelling, naturally purifying options for homemade cleaning recipes. Add oils to green your laundry routine, sanitize the kitchen, and nix mold in the bathroom, all while making your house smell clean—no scary fumes needed! I'm inclined to add lemon, grapefruit, tea tree, and lavender to just about every cleaning recipe, but there are lots more you might want to have on hand.

First, let's talk about citrus essential oils and their main chemical constituent, limonene. Most citrus essential oils have some form of limonene in them, which is a powerful antioxidant and cleansing agent. The ancient Egyptians used to use lemon essential oil to remove toxins from their bodies. Limonene also can dissolve oils, making it ideal for a variety of cleaning purposes. That said, it can also eat into plastic, causing toxins to escape into the contents of a spray bottle or water bottle, so I always recommend using glass to store your cleaning products. You can even do a simple test to see the power of citrus essential oil: Have a pesky sticker that won't come off or left an adhesive residue behind? Put a drop of lemon oil on it, rub it in, and then wipe it away. It is like magic—all-natural magic!

Now, when you combine that grease-fighting ability with white vinegar, you have a match made in heaven. White vinegar contains natural antifungal and antibacterial properties. It also has an amazing ability to cut into grease, especially mineral deposits like lime scale from hard water or that nasty toilet ring. Here are some essential cleaning tips:

FRESHEN THE LAUNDRY: Add lavender, lemon, or melaleuca essential oil to the washing machine during the wash cycle. Essential oils will brighten and disinfect clothing. Clove, lemon, and eucalyptus in the rinse cycle are great for ridding towels of environmental threats.

VACUUMING: If you have a bag vacuum, add many drops of oil to a disposable cloth or tissue and place in the collecting bag. With a water reservoir, add a few drops before cleaning and the oil will diffuse around the room. Use clean, distilled water, which acts as a carrier and dirt solvent. Tap water often contains salts and minerals that can lead to spotting and buildup.

DISHWASHING: For very greasy dishes, add ⅓ cup distilled white vinegar and 5 drops of lemon essential oil to dishwater. To loosen baked-on food from pots and pans, boil 2 cups water, 5 drops of lemon essential oil, and 3 tablespoons of baking soda and add directly in the pot or pan. Allow mixture to stand until food can be easily scraped off the surface.

AIR PURIFICATION: To lessen indoor pollutants, diffuse citrus oils throughout the house. Lemon and grapefruit are great options.

Below you will find my top green cleaning recipes and a shopping list of key ingredients for making your easy, homemade cleaning products.

- Essential oils (lemon, grape-fruit, melaleuca, lavender, orange, eucalyptus)
- Baking soda
- Liquid Castile soap (Dr. Bronner's unscented liquid soap)
- White distilled vinegar
- Olive or almond oil
- Distilled water
- Kosher salt
- Apple cider vinegar
- Rubbing alcohol
- Bowls
- Spray bottles
- Soft cotton dusting cloth
- Vegetable glycerin
- Natural bristle scrubbing brushes
- Tote bag (for carrying cleaning supplies)
- Washing soda

Household Cleaning Recipes

AIR FRESHENER SPRAY

This spray is great as a daily home freshener. Your home says something special and unique about you. Create a special scent that your family and friends can enjoy. Get creative and mix and match essential oils. Another combination that I love includes grapefruit, rosemary, and ylang ylang.

YIELD: 8-ounce spray bottle

¾ cup water
6 drops lavender essential oil
6 drops lemon essential oil
3 drops peppermint essential oil

DIRECTIONS: Combine the water and essential oils in an 8-ounce glass spray bottle and spray 3 to 4 times in each room of the house.

STICKER OR GUM REMOVER

Lemon essential oil is great at removing sticky and greasy residue.

YIELD: 1 to 2 applications

1 teaspoon baking soda
1 teaspoon almond oil or olive oil
3 drops lemon essential oil

DIRECTIONS: Mix all of the ingredients in a small bowl. Apply a small amount to the sticker or gum and let sit for 1 to 2 minutes. Use a soft cloth to remove the sticky substance on the area. Continue to apply, if needed, until sticky spot is removed.

CARPET FRESHENER

YIELD: 8 to 10 applications

2 cups baking soda
10 drops lavender essential oil

DIRECTIONS: Combine the baking soda and lavender essential oil in a mason jar. Cap and shake well to combine. Remove cap and replace inner lid with construction paper. Secure rim and cut off excess construction paper. Poke holes in the construction paper. Apply carpet freshener liberally to carpets. Wait 1 to 2 hours. Vacuum over carpet thoroughly.

DUSTING AND CLEANING CLOTH FOR WOOD

YIELD: 1 application

⅓ teaspoon olive oil

¼ cup vinegar

4 drops lemon essential oil

DIRECTIONS: Mix all of the ingredients together and add to cleaning cloth. Dab soft cloth on wood surfaces to polish wood. Reuse cloth for other wood surfaces up to six times.

NATURAL SCRATCH REMOVER

YIELD: 1 application

1 tablespoon lemon juice

1 teaspoon distilled white vinegar

3 to 5 drops lemon essential oil

DIRECTIONS: Mix all of the ingredients in a small bowl. Dip soft cloth into mixture and gently rub onto wood surface scratch. Rub on scratches until they disappear. For deeper scratches, rub in mixture until they shrink in size. Buff away any remaining residue with a dry soft cloth.

BASIC HARDWOOD AND CERAMIC TILE FLOOR CLEANER

YIELD: 1 application

1 gallon hot water

¼ cup Castile liquid soap

¼ cup distilled white vinegar

10 drops melaleuca essential oil

DIRECTIONS: Mix water, Castile soap, vinegar, and essential oil in a large bucket. Mop with a dry mop or scrub with a microfiber cloth by hand. Change cleaning solution as needed.

VINYL FLOOR CLEANSER

This cleaner is for stubborn stains, such as permanent marker. Increase concentration by adding more isopropyl alcohol. This cleaner can also be used on tile, linoleum, and marble.

YIELD: 1 application

4 cups hot water

1 teaspoon liquid dish soap

1 cup distilled white vinegar

1 cup isopropyl alcohol (rubbing alcohol)

10 drops lemon essential oil

DIRECTIONS: Mix water, dish soap, vinegar, isopropyl alcohol, and essential oil in a large bowl. Mop with a dry mop or scrub with microfiber cloth by hand. Change cleaning solution as needed.

CARPET STAIN REMOVER

YIELD: 1 application

3 cups water, divided

1 tablespoon Castile liquid soap

10 drops lemon essential oil

DIRECTIONS: Mix half of the water, the Castile soap, and the essential oil into a bowl. Soak a soft cloth in the mixture, wring it out, and gently blot the stain. Use a clean, dry, soft cloth and soak it in the remaining clean water to remove the residue. Continue to alternate between the soap solution and the clean water until the stain is not visible.

Note: Remember to blot, not rub, the carpet or upholstery stain so you do not damage the fabric or fibers.

Kitchen Cleaning Recipes

FOAMING HAND SOAP

Foaming hand soap is great for every bathroom and kitchen. Essential oil recommendations are melaleuca, lavender, orange, peppermint, eucalyptus, and grapefruit.

YIELD: 8- to 12-ounce bottle

3 tablespoons liquid Castile soap

½ teaspoon almond oil

10 drops essential oil of choice

1 to 2 cups water

DIRECTIONS: Combine Castile soap and almond oil in a bottle with a foaming pump. Add essential oil of your choice. Slowly add water to the bottle, leaving space for the pump to screw into the bottle. Shake gently before using.

LIQUID DISH SOAP

YIELD: 20-ounce dish soap squirt bottle or pump dispenser

2 cups unscented liquid Castile soap

½ cup warm water

5 drops lime essential oil

5 drops orange essential oil

DIRECTIONS: Fill the dish soap container with Castile soap, warm water, and essential oils. Shake container and use on dishes.

OVEN CLEANER PASTE

YIELD: 1 application

2 cups baking soda

1 cup water

2 tablespoons Castile soap

15 drops lemon essential oil

DIRECTIONS: Combine all of the ingredients in a small bowl to form a thick paste. Use more baking soda to increase thickness as desired. Apply paste with a sponge and let sit for 30 minutes. Wipe off with clean cloth, or with a sponge and water.

TRASH CAN DEODORIZING TABLETS

You can also use these tablets in the refrigerator, under the sink, in a shoe closet, or any place in the house you want to deodorize.

YIELD: 6 to 8 tablets

2 cups baking soda

1 to 2 cups distilled water

5 drops peppermint

5 drops grapefruit

DIRECTIONS: Add the baking soda to a bowl. In a separate small bowl, combine the water and essential oils and add them to the baking soda by slowly stirring to achieve the desired paste. Transfer mixture into silicone molds or a muffin pan and allow to dry overnight, or until the tablets have hardened. Place 1 to 2 tablets into trash cans throughout the house. The tablets are good for 30 days. Store unused tablets in an airtight container.

Note: When you are ready to replace it, take the OLD tablet and crumble it into a load of laundry to help deodorize there as well.

AUTOMATIC DISHWASHING POWDER

YIELD: 24 loads

3 cups washing soda

15 drops lemon or lime essential oil

1 cup baking soda

DIRECTIONS: Combine all ingredients and store in a sealed container. To use, add approximately 2 tablespoons to the soap compartment of your dishwasher. If the glasses start to accumulate residue, decrease to 1½ tablespoons of powder.

FRUIT AND VEGETABLE WASH

It's important to wash pesticides and environmental threats from your produce. This wash will remove all of the residues from your fruits and vegetables.

YIELD: 1 wash

4 cups filtered water

1 cup apple cider vinegar

10 drops lemon essential oil

DIRECTIONS: In a large bowl mix filtered water, vinegar, and essential oil. To use, submerge produce in the bowl. Stir the produce around with your hand to make sure all of the produce comes in contact with the lemon essential oil. Let the produce sit for 30 to 60 seconds. Rinse with filtered water in a strainer.

Bathroom Cleaning Recipes

TOILET AND TUB SOFT SCRUB CLEANER

YIELD: 2 applications

1 cup baking soda

10 drops melaleuca essential oil

1 teaspoon vegetable glycerin

½ cup unscented liquid Castile soap

DIRECTIONS: Add baking soda, essential oil, and vegetable glycerin to a bowl and slowly add the Castile soap until a paste is formed.

TO USE: Apply the soft scrub paste to soap scum in bathtubs, toilet bowls, and sinks. Let sit for 10 to 15 minutes. Scrub will with a brush or sponge and rinse off.

HOMEMADE BATHROOM CLEANING POWDER

Great for bathtubs, showers, and kitchen and bathroom sinks.

YIELD: 10 to 12 applications

2 cups borax

1 cup baking soda

¾ cup kosher salt

10 drops melaleuca essential oil

10 drops lemon essential oil

DIRECTIONS: Combine all of the ingredients into a Mason jar or other shaker bottle. I recommend using an empty large spice container.

TO USE: Dampen the surface area with water or vinegar and sprinkle the cleaning powder over the area. Let sit for 10 to 15 minutes and scrub with a sponge or brush. Rinse clean.

MULTIPLE-PURPOSE CLEANING SPRAY

YIELD: 12-ounce spray bottle

1 cup distilled white vinegar

2 cups distilled water

5 drops melaleuca essential oil

5 drops lemon essential oil

DIRECTIONS: Add all ingredients to a 12-ounce spray bottle and shake well. Use as you would any other all-purpose cleaner for countertops, porcelain surfaces, mirrors, tile, and other household surfaces. Wipe with a microfiber cloth or clean sponge. If unsure of whether this should be used on a certain surface area, test the cleaner on a small area first.

Note: For tougher areas of the house, leave the spray solution on that surface for 30 minutes before rinsing.

MOLD AND SCUM PREVENTION SPRAY

YIELD: 12-ounce spray bottle

3 cups water

1 tablespoon rubbing alcohol

25 drops melaleuca essential oil

10 drops eucalyptus essential oil

DIRECTIONS: Add all ingredients to the spray bottle and shake well. Spray directly on mold or scum buildup in the shower, tub, or anywhere else in the bathroom. Do not rinse. Repeat daily or weekly as needed.

WINDOW AND MIRROR SPRAY CLEANER

YIELD: 16-ounce spray bottle

3 cups distilled water

3 tablespoons distilled white vinegar

2 tablespoons rubbing alcohol

5 drops lemon or grapefruit essential oil

DIRECTIONS: Add all ingredients into a spray bottle and shake well. Spray windows and mirrors and wipe down with microfiber cloth, newspaper, or paper towels. Store unused solution for up to 2 to 3 months.

Laundry Cleaning Recipes

LAUNDRY STAIN REMOVER

This is a great cleaning solution for greasy and stubborn stains, such as blood and grass stains.

YIELD: 8-ounce glass spray bottle

2 cups distilled white vinegar

25 drops lemon essential oil

DIRECTIONS: Combined ingredients in the spray bottle and shake well. Spray solution on the stain, let sit for 5 to 10 minutes, and wash.

DIY DRYER SOFTENER BALLS

YIELD: 4 to 6 dryer balls

1 skein 100% wool yarn

pantyhose

6 to 8 drops lavender, bergamot orange, or lemon essential oil per dryer ball

DIRECTIONS: Take the end of the wool yarn and wrap it around your index and middle finger 10 to 15 times. Next, remove the yarn from the 2 fingers and then wrap 2 or 3 times around the middle. It should look like a little bow. Continue to tightly wrap the yarn around, making a round shape the size of a tennis ball. Once the size of the tennis ball, cut the ends and tuck them into the ball. Repeat the directions for 3 to 5 more balls.

Cut one leg off the pantyhose. Place one yarn ball into the bottom of the pantyhose and tie a tight knot above the ball to secure the shape of the ball. Repeat until all of the balls have been added and secured. Once all of the yarn balls are secured, then wash and dry them on the highest heat setting in the dryer.

When the dryer balls are completely dry, remove the pantyhose and add 6 to 8 drops of your favorite essential oil to each ball. For best results, toss 4 to 6 balls into dryer with clothes.

LIQUID FABRIC SOFTENER

YIELD: 18 loads

½ gallon distilled white vinegar

1 cup baking soda

30 drops lavender essential oil

DIRECTIONS: Combine ingredients into 1 large storage container and add ½ cup to each load of laundry in the washer. The laundry will soften and smell great, too.

LAUNDRY SOAP RECIPE

YIELD: 24 to 48 loads, depending on the size of load

1 finely grated bar baby mild unscented Castile soap

1 cup washing soda

1 cup borax

10 drops lemon essential oil

10 drops grapefruit or wild orange essential oil

DIRECTIONS: Mix grated Castile soap, washing soda, and borax together in a bowl with a spoon. Add essential oils and stir completely. Store in sealed, airtight glass jar. Use 1 to 2 tablespoons per load, depending on size of the load.

Note: This recipe is safe for high-efficiency washers. For extra-dirty loads of laundry, consider adding an oxygen booster to the washer along with this recipe.

CHAPTER

NATURAL PERSONAL AND BEAUTY CARE RECIPES

When it comes to keeping the entire family safe from harmful chemicals and damaging endocrine disruptors, it's important to start reading labels on everything that will come into contact with the body, especially the skin, the body's largest organ. It's not enough to only focus on what you put into your mouth. Chemical exposure through daily personal care products is a reality that you must address in order to keep the entire family healthy.

According to the Environmental Working Group (EWG), the average woman applies 168 chemicals from 10 to 12 skincare products to her skin daily. Since your skin acts more like a sponge than a barrier, those chemicals are absorbed into the body.

There is now strong scientific evidence linking dangerous toxins and synthetics in personal care products to chronic diseases, reproductive toxicity, autoimmunity, allergies, and cancer. Recent studies have found that parabens and phthalates from fragrances, cosmetics, and even shampoos are showing up in breast milk and body tissues. Equally as important is the impact synthetic preservatives and fragrances are having on our environment. Persistent pollutants do not degrade; instead, they remain in our water supply and soil. This in turn affects our food and water supply.

Unfortunately, the Food and Drug Administration (FDA) and cosmetic corporations maintain that these chemicals are safe in small doses. But when you consider that the average family uses shampoo, lotion, cleansers, and hand wash every day, you begin to understand how toxins begin to add up over time. Almost 90 percent of the 10,000+ cosmetics and skincare ingredients known to the FDA have not been evaluated for safety by any publicly accountable institution, including the FDA, according to the EWG.

As a hormone expert, I have studied the effects of synthetic chemicals on endocrine and reproductive health. The endocrine system is your hormone regulating system, regulating everything from reproduction, mood, and immunity to metabolism and brain function. Xenoestrogens such as BPA, parabens, and phthalates can alter female reproductive development and fertility and influence metabolism, mood, and the early onset of menopause. In men, these chemicals are linked to male infertility, cancer, and even genital deformities. Children are even more susceptible to endocrine disruptors, as their bodies are not fully developed. Brain, reproductive, and metabolic development have shown to be negatively affected by endocrine disruptors.

As I mentioned above, becoming label savvy is very important to choosing the right natural products for the whole family. However, there are thousands of ingredients out there that may make it more challenging to read the labels of your beauty and personal care products. This is why I recommend making as many as your own natural personal care products as possible. Luckily, everyday products are very simple and cost effective to make, especially when harnessing the power of therapeutic essential oils. I have compiled a comparable list of recipes with nourishing ingredients found in grocery and natural health food stores. These recipes are easy to make and cost a fraction of the price of store-bought counterparts.

The natural ingredients in these recipes are enhanced by the many therapeutic benefits of essential oils. Essential oils are truly a gift from the earth when it comes to nourishing the skin, hair, and nails; that's why they have been used in personal care products and cosmetics for hundreds of years. The many chemical constituents contained in essential oils are designed to provide nourishing benefits to the body inside and out. Specifically, essentials oils are great for soothing skin and supporting cellular regeneration. Essential oils can support healthy antiaging through promoting new cell growth, toning skin, and reducing blemishes and wrinkles. They are also effective at addressing chapped, dry skin, such as on hands and feet.

Essential oils such as helichrysum, sandalwood, and rose are effective for reducing the appearance of blemishes and creating more radiant, youthful skin. The chemical properties in lavender, melaleuca, frankincense and Roman chamomile are very safe on children and ideal for sensitive skin.

Geranium is a Swiss army knife when it comes to providing tools for the skin. Paired with lavender, common skin irritations are quickly resolved.

Citrus essential oils are great for toning and purifying the body along with providing immune and mood support. Citrus oils also contain unique photosensitive compounds called furocoumarins. Be sure to avoid exposure to direct sunlight or other sources of UV light for up to 10 to 12 hours after topically applying these essential oils to the skin.

The recipes in this section are safe for children three years and older. Many of the recipes are also safe for younger children, but I would consider only using 5 to 8 drops per recipe to be safe. Many of the carrier oils are also very safe, but each person's skin is different, so spot test the recipes before applying to the face or sensitive areas of the body.

Spa Recipes

EUCALYPTUS SUGAR SCRUB

Eucalyptus oil will give your skin a nice, clean, tingling sensation. Eucalyptus is perfect for relieving muscle tension and providing a soothing skin massage experience. Other oils to consider for homemade sugar scrubs are orange, grapefruit, lavender, and peppermint. Add more oil for a wetter consistency.

YIELD: 2 jars

3 cups organic turbinado sugar

2 cups almond oil or fractionated coconut oil

10 drops eucalyptus essential oil

DIRECTIONS: In a mixing bowl, add the sugar and the almond or coconut oil. Add the eucalyptus essential oil and mix it in thoroughly. Spoon the scrub mixture into the glass jars and store at room temperature. Apply scrub during the shower for soft, healthy skin.

CHAMOMILE LAVENDER OATMEAL MILK BATH

The dry milk in this recipe provides softening benefits for all skin types. Oatmeal is naturally soothing for sensitive skin. Lavender and Roman chamomile are both known for their calming aromatherapy benefits, so they are perfect partners for this milk bath. Other essential oils to consider are geranium, rose, and jasmine.

YIELD: about 3 cups

2 cups dried milk

½ cup baking soda

½ cup ground oats

8 drops Roman chamomile essential oil

8 drops lavender essential oil

¼ cup dry lavender flowers

DIRECTIONS: Stir dried milk, baking soda, and ground oats together. Add the essential oils and stir together. Next, stir in the lavender flowers. Divide oatmeal milk bath into 3 small glass mason jars.

FOR YOUR BATH: Add approximately ¼ to ½ cup of the oatmeal milk bath to warm water and stir to dissolve. The lavender flowers will soften a bit and float during the bath. Remember to remove them before draining the bath tub.

FOAMING HAND SOAP

Foaming hand soap is great for every bathroom and kitchen. Essential oil recommendations are melaleuca, lavender, orange, peppermint, eucalyptus, and grapefruit.

YIELD: 8- to 12-ounce bottle with foam pump

3 tablespoons liquid Castile soap

½ teaspoon almond oil

10 drops essential oil of choice

1 to 2 cups water

DIRECTIONS: Combine Castile soap and almond oil into a bottle with foaming pump. Add essential oil of your choice. Slowly add water to bottle, leaving space for the foaming pump to screw into the bottle. Shake gently before using.

HOMEMADE CITRUS BODY BUTTER

Apply homemade body butter after your morning shower for soft and invigorated skin. Lime and orange essential oils are perfect for toning skin and energizing the senses.

YIELD: 12-ounce container

1 cup unrefined shea butter

½ cup coconut oil

½ cup almond oil

20 drops lime essential oil

10 drops orange essential oil

DIRECTIONS: Heat shea butter, coconut oil, and almond oil together over a double boiler. Cool mixture to room temperature and add essential oils. Next, refrigerate mixture for an hour or so. Once solid, whip with mixing beaters until smooth. Store in a glass or stainless steel container.

REJUVENATING PINK SALT SCRUB

Eucalyptus oil will give your skin a nice tingling sensation. I chose geranium and chamomile to relieve, soften, and nourish the skin. Other oils to consider for homemade salt scrubs are ginger, lime, orange, lavender, and frankincense. Add more coconut or almond oil for a wetter consistency.

YIELD: 12-ounce container

2 cups ground Himalayan salt

1 cup grape-seed oil

1 cup fractionated coconut oil or almond oil

10 drops geranium essential oil

10 drops chamomile essential oil

DIRECTIONS: In a mixing bowl, add the Himalayan salt. Mix in the grape-seed oil and almond or coconut oil. Add the essential oils and mix in thoroughly. Next, spoon scrub mixture into a glass jar and store at room temperature. Apply salt scrub during the shower for soft, healthy skin.

GENTLE AND RELAXING BUBBLE BATH

The bubbles in this recipe are not mountainous bubbles, and they don't last a long time. But they do provide enough bubbles for your children to play in and for you to have a relaxing bath experience. The ingredients are very easy to find in any health food store. Lavender, wild orange, and a touch of ylang ylang provide a calming and aromatic bubble bath for everyone in the family to enjoy. Other essential oils to consider for a relaxing bubble bath are lavender, frankincense, jasmine, Roman chamomile, and clary sage.

YIELD: 8-ounce glass container

1 cup unscented baby mild Castile soap

⅓ cup vegetable glycerin

3 tablespoons white sugar

5 drops lavender essential oil

5 drops wild orange essential oil

2 drops ylang ylang essential oil

DIRECTIONS: In a small glass bowl, combine Castile soap, vegetable glycerin, sugar, and essential oils. Stir mixture until well combined. Pour bubble bath solution into a glass container and let sit for at least 12 hours before using. For a bubble bath, add ⅛ cup of the bubble bath mixture to warm or hot running water.

Personal Skin and Hair Care Recipes

CHOCOLATE ORANGE AND PEPPERMINT LIP BALM

YIELD: 2 lip balm tubes or containers

5 tablespoons coconut oil

3 tablespoons beeswax

6 drops orange essential oil

6 drops peppermint essential oil

¼ teaspoon cocoa powder

DIRECTIONS: Add coconut oil and beeswax into a glass measuring cup. Melt the coconut oil and beeswax in a double boiler. Once the mixture is clear and completely melted, stir in the essential oils and cocoa powder. Mix all the ingredients together and pour into the empty lip balm tubes or containers. Apply on chapped lips to moisturize and soften.

JASMINE AND HONEY FACE WASH

This face wash is very gentle and designed for all skin types, especially combination skin. Feel free to play with ingredient amounts for your skin type. For example, for drier skin types, use less Castile soap and vegetable glycerin and more jojoba oil. Jasmine essential oil is perfect for creating balanced skin and melaleuca is designed to keep the skin free of impurities. Other essential oils to consider for a face wash are rosemary, lavender, geranium, frankincense, and rose.

YIELD: 8-ounce glass container

½ cup filtered water

¼ cup unscented baby mild Castile soap

2 tablespoons organic raw honey

3 teaspoons jojoba oil

1 teaspoon vitamin E

1 teaspoon vegetable glycerin

15 drops jasmine essential oil

5 drops melaleuca essential oil

DIRECTIONS: In a small bowl, add the water then mix in all other ingredients. Gently whisk together until completely integrated. Pour face wash into a liquid soap dispenser. Use 1 to 2 pumps with a little water and apply to face with gentle circular motions. Rinse with cool water and pat dry.

CLEAR COMPLEXION BLEMISH ROLLERBALL BLEND

Black cumin seed and melaleuca reduce breakouts and clear up skin impurities. Lavender, rosemary, and lemon promote a clear complexion while being gentle on the skin. Skin will feel smoother, cleaner, and more hydrated.

YIELD: 10-ounce rollerball bottle

15 drops melaleuca essential oil

15 black cumin seed essential oil

10 drops lavender essential oil

5 drops rosemary essential oil

5 drops lemon essential oil

Fractionated coconut oil

DIRECTIONS: Add essential oil to the empty rollerball bottle, then top off the remainder of the rollerball bottle with fractionated coconut oil. Attach the rollerball to the bottle, close the lid, and gently turn rollerball bottle up and down approximately 15 times, until blend is completely mixed together. Apply blemish blend to affected areas of the skin, morning and night, after washing and drying face.

POST-SUN SOOTHING SPRAY

Coconut oil, witch hazel, and pure aloe vera are wonderful for hydrating irritated skin. Lavender essential oil is known as the best calming oil, especially for irritated skin, and peppermint essential oil is perfect to cool skin down. You can find aloe vera at any health food store.

YIELD: 8-ounce glass spray bottle

½ cup witch hazel

3 tablespoons pure aloe vera gel

¼ cup fractionated coconut oil

1 teaspoon vitamin E

10 drops lavender essential oil

6 drops peppermint essential oil

DIRECTIONS: Combine all ingredients in a glass spray bottle and shake the bottle until they are mixed completely together. Spray over irritated skin every hour to soothe.

AGE-DEFIANT FACE CREAM

Frankincense and lavender are amazing for antiaging skin properties, along with reducing the appearance of skin imperfections. The facial cream is very versatile. Feel free to experiment with different essential oil, hydrosol, and oil combinations to see which combination works best for your skin. Other essential oils to consider are sandalwood, helichrysum, rose, jasmine, orange, and geranium.

If this cream is too rich for your face, you can use it for your hands and feet instead to sooth dry, cracked skin. Essential oils to consider for hand

and foot creams are peppermint, rose geranium, calendula, lemon, and eucalyptus.

YIELD: 5 (4-ounce) containers

¼ cup organic olive oil

¼ cup organic sweet almond oil

¼ cup organic apricot oil

1 tablespoon organic coconut oil

1 tablespoon beeswax pastilles or carnauba wax (vegan option)

1 cup organic rose, rose geranium, or helichrysum hydrosol

½ cup organic aloe vera gel

¼ teaspoon vitamin E oil (a punctured capsule should be perfect)

8 drops frankincense essential oil

5 drops lavender essential oil

DIRECTIONS: Blend oils together in a double boiler on very low heat, just enough to thoroughly warm. Once warm, add in the beeswax pastilles or carnauba wax and gently whisk until they've completely dissolved into the oil mixture. Next, pour the hydrosol, aloe vera gel, vitamin E, and essential oils into your blender. Turn the blender on low and slowly add the warmed oil mixture into the center of the blender in a slow, steady stream. It all has to be mixed together completely to ensure that the cream emulsifies properly and doesn't clump up. Use your spatula to scrape the edges. This will scoop up any unmixed bits and ensure the creamy texture. Once you've done this, turn the blender on low to finish mixing the cream.

Use a spatula to scrape the cream out of the blender and use a spoon to decant into the empty jars. Lid and label the jars with a date and the essential oils that you used. Keep the extra jars in the refrigerator to last longer. This cream can last 6 to 10 months stored in the refrigerator. Always smell it, or look for mold to ensure it's still fresh.

TINTED PEPPERMINT LIP GLOSS

Peppermint essential oil adds a slight tingle to the lip gloss, so feel free to adjust the number of drops depending on how much tingle you prefer.

If you prefer to make a couple of different essential oil combinations from this batch, you can pour some of the mixture into different spouted measuring cups and add the essential oils separately, or you can just flavor the whole batch as this recipe suggests.

Other essential oil combinations to try are grapefruit and vanilla, peppermint and wild orange, and lime and lemon. When combining essential oils, play with the number of drops. Some essential oils are stronger in smell and taste than other ones. Dab a little of the mixture onto your lips to test out the concentration, but note that the flavors and scents will get a bit stronger when the gloss hardens.

YIELD: 8 (1-ounce) containers

¾ cup organic refined coconut oil (unscented)
¼ teaspoon vitamin E oil (or 1 big capsule)
¼ cup beeswax pastilles
10 to 15 drops peppermint essential oil
¼ teaspoon pigment, such as hibiscus flower powder or beet root powder (optional)

DIRECTIONS: Blend oils together in a double boiler and stir gently. Next, add in the beeswax pastilles and gently whisk until they've completely dissolved into the oil mixture. Turn off heat and add peppermint essential oil and pigment, stirring with a small spoon combine. If mixture begins to thicken before pouring into gloss tubes, turn the heat back to low.

With a dropper, fill lip gloss tubes with mixture. Let the tubes set for 15 to 20 minutes.

HOT OIL HAIR TREATMENT

Rosemary and lavender essential oil promotes strong and healthy hair. Repeat hot oil treatment 2 to 3 times a month for thicker, healthier, and shiny hair.

YIELD: 1 application

2 cups water
1 tablespoon avocado oil

2 tablespoons coconut oil

1 teaspoon olive oil

5 drops lavender essential oil

4 drops rosemary essential oil

DIRECTIONS: In a small sauce pan, bring the water to a boil. Reduce heat to low. Place all ingredients except for essential oils in a heat-resistant bowl and let the hot oil mixture heat up for 5 minutes. Remove the bowl from heat and add the lavender and rosemary essential oils, gently stirring with a spoon or fingers.

To apply, dip your fingertips into the oil mixture and gently massage oil from the scalp to the ends of hair. Once hair is thoroughly coated, wrap in a towel or shower cap for 30 minutes. After treatment, shampoo and condition hair.

HOMEMADE NATURAL DEODORANT

Melaleuca is great for reducing odor-causing bacteria. Bergamot is a clean citrus essential oil that acts as a natural deodorant and has skin purifying benefits. Other recommended essential oils are lavender, lime, geranium, thyme, and frankincense.

YIELD: 2½-ounce deodorant container

¼ cup baking soda

¼ cup arrowroot powder

5 drops melaleuca essential oil

5 drops bergamot or grapefruit essential oil

4 tablespoons organic unrefined coconut oil, melted

DIRECTIONS: In a bowl, stir together the dry ingredients and the essential oils. Slowly add one tablespoon of coconut oil at a time, mixing well to achieve desired consistency. Store in a shallow, airtight container, or press firmly into an empty deodorant container. Let sit until completely solidified. Apply a small amount to the underarm area to keep dry.

Note: If you live in a hot climate, consider adding ½ teaspoon of beeswax to recipe.

SOOTHING SALVE

You may use this salve as a base for various health applications. Add eucalyptus and peppermint for respiratory support. Add lavender and chamomile for relaxing muscle tension. Add orange and lime for invigorating the senses. This salve is also great for tired, chapped feet and hands.

YIELD: 8-ounce glass container

2 tablespoons beeswax

½ cup grape seed oil

½ cup fractionated coconut oil or almond oil

2 teaspoons vitamin E oil

10 drops frankincense essential oil

5 drops lavender essential oil

5 drops melaleuca essential oil

DIRECTIONS: Melt the beeswax in a double boiler. Once melted, add the grape-seed oil, coconut or almond oil, and vitamin E oil and melt everything down. Once ingredients are combined, set aside for 4 to 5 minutes. Next, add essential oils and stir completely. Pour mixture into glass container and let sit for 1 to 2 hours. Apply soothing salve to skin.

INVIGORATING EXFOLIATING SCRUB

Exfoliating your face will help to slough away dry skin, leaving your face much softer and smoother. This recipe takes about 5 minutes to make, and the scrub can be used twice a week. Lime essential oil provides added cleaning and clarifying properties. Feel free to also use wild orange, geranium, and frankincense.

YIELD: 1 application

2 tablespoons ground oatmeal

⅓ teaspoon ground sea salt

2 teaspoon water

½ teaspoon coconut oil

2 drops lime essential oil

½ teaspoon honey

DIRECTIONS: Combine all ingredients in a small bowl and stir until a paste is formed. If you find that it's too thick, add a bit more water or coconut oil until it reaches the desired consistency. Slather it on your face and use your fingertips to rub it around gently in upward, circular motions. Rinse with warm (not hot) water, and pat dry.

DRY SHAMPOO

YIELD: 4-ounce jar

LIGHT HAIR
½ cup arrowroot powder
3 drops rosemary essential oil
5 drops lavender essential oil

DARK HAIR
3 tablespoons arrowroot powder
3 drops rosemary essential oil
5 drops lavender essential oil
3 tablespoons cocoa powder

DIRECTIONS: Add arrowroot powder, essential oils, and cocoa powder (for the dark hair recipe) into a mixing bowl. Mix with electric mixer until completely combined. Store dry shampoo in a glass jar or old powder container. Apply to roots with a makeup brush.

RICH COCONUT OIL HAIR MASK

Cedarwood and lavender essential oils promote strong and healthy hair while relieving dry scalp. Coconut and raw honey penetrate the hair shaft and moisturize from within to repair dry and damaged hair. Coconut will also protect from future damage. Repeat coconut mask treatment 2 to 3 times a month for healthier, shinier hair.

YIELD: 1 application
2 cups water
⅛ cup coconut oil
2 tablespoons raw honey

1 tablespoon apple cider vinegar

3 drops cedarwood essential oil

3 drops lavender essential oil

DIRECTIONS: In a medium sauce pan, bring water to a boil. Reduce heat to low. Place heat-resistant bowl in sauce pan. Add coconut oil and honey to the heat-resistant bowl and mix together. Remove the bowl from the sauce pan, add apple cider vinegar and essential oils, and gently stir with a spoon.

The best way to apply the mask is to use a coloring brush. Section your hair into 3 equal parts. Apply the coconut oil mask from the root down to the tips of your hair. Be sure to massage the oil into the scalp as well. Once hair is thoroughly coated, pile into a bun and leave for 20 to 30 minutes. After treatment, shampoo and condition hair.

DIY NATURAL SHAMPOO

YIELD: 12-ounce glass dispenser

1 cup liquid Castile soap

½ cup canned or homemade coconut milk

⅛ cup raw honey

2 tablespoons fractionated coconut oil

10 drops lavender essential oil

6 drops peppermint essential oil

6 drops wild orange essential oil

DIRECTIONS: Mix all of the ingredients in a squeeze bottle or glass dispenser. Shake bottle before using and applying to hair.

NATURAL DIY CONDITIONER

YIELD: 8-ounce spray bottle

1½ cups of water

3 tablespoons organic apple cider vinegar

6 drops rosemary essential oil

3 drops lemon essential oil

3 drops bergamot essential oil

DIRECTIONS: Add all ingredients into a spray bottle. Shake bottle before using and working into hair.

SOLID HOMEMADE PERFUME

YIELD: 1 application

1 tablespoon beeswax

3 tablespoons grape-seed oil

1 tablespoon almond oil

20 drops essential oil blend

1 metal container (to store perfume)

DIRECTIONS: Melt the beeswax in a double boiler. Add grape-seed and almond oils and stir ingredients completely, approximately 1 to 3 minutes. Once melted, remove from heat and let sit for 3 to 5 minutes. Add essential oil blend to mixture and stir.

Pour perfume blend into a metal container and let harden for 10 to 15 minutes. Store in purse for easy access.

Note: I recommend adorning yourself with your favorite perfume throughout the day for incredible aromatherapy and mood benefits. I have included some of my favorite perfume blends below to use for this recipe.

ESSENTIAL OIL PERFUME BLENDS

YIELD: 1 application

LIGHT AND WISTFUL BLEND

5 drops lavender

5 drops cedarwood

7 drops clary sage

3 drops ylang ylang

SELF-LOVE BLEND
8 drops lavender

8 drops bergamot

4 drops ylang ylang

SWEET AND ENERGIZING BLEND
7 drops grapefruit

6 drops ginger

4 drops vetiver

3 drops lime

SENSUAL AND WARM BLEND
8 drops sandalwood

5 drops wild orange

4 drops vetiver

3 drops ylang ylang

SOOTHING HOMEMADE SHAVING CREAM

This shaving cream can be used for both men and women alike. It acts as a great moisturizer, so there's no need to use a lotion or body butter after shaving. Peppermint and grapefruit essential oils are energizing and smell incredible together. Also try wild orange and lime, or lavender and bergamot.

YIELD: 12-ounce glass container

1 cup shea butter

1 cup cold-pressed coconut oil

½ cup jojoba oil

7 drops grapefruit essential oil

5 drops peppermint essential oil

1 tablespoon vitamin E oil

DIRECTIONS: Heat shea butter and coconut oil together over a double boiler. Take the mixture off the heat for 3 to 5 minutes and add jojoba, essential oils, and vitamin E oil. Cool mixture to room temperature. Next, refrigerate mixture for an hour or so. Once solid, whip with mixing beaters until completely smooth. Store in a 12-ounce glass or stainless steel container with lid.

LAVENDER-COCOA BODY LOTION BARS

This is the easiest lotion recipe that you are going to find. Feel free to play with the molds and give them as gifts. Other essential oils that nourish the skin and are great to combine are lavender and frankincense, jasmine and sandalwood, clary sage and cedarwood, and rosemary and lavender.

YIELD: 10 to 12 bars (depending on molds)

1 cup beeswax pastilles

1 cup cocoa butter

1 cup coconut oil

2 teaspoons vitamin E

10 drops lavender essential oil

10 drops geranium essential oil

DIRECTIONS: Combine all ingredients except essential oils in a double boiler or a glass bowl over a smaller sauce pan with 1 inch of water in it. Bring to a boil. Stir ingredients until they are completely melted and smooth. Remove from heat and then add essential oils. Stir to incorporate essential oils. Pour mixture into silicone baking cup molds for the lotion to solidify. Allow the lotion bars to completely dry before removing them from the molds. Store lotion bars in a clean container and apply to body after a shower. The heat from your body will melt the lotion.

MOISTURIZING HAND CREAM

This recipe is a thicker version of the facial cream and ideal for chapped, dry hands. You can even try this recipe on your feet. Wild orange and ylang ylang provide a calm and uplifting effect when applied to skin. Suggested essential oils for conditioning skin are helichrysum, lavender, frankincense, sandalwood, rose, chamomile, and geranium.

YIELD: 5 (4-ounce) jars

¼ cup almond oil

¼ cup jojoba oil

⅛ cocoa butter

½ cup fractionated coconut oil

1 tablespoon beeswax or carnauba wax pastilles

½ cup calendula or rose hydrosol

½ teaspoon vitamin E

10 drops wild orange essential oil

5 drops ylang ylang essential oil

DIRECTIONS: Blend oils and cocoa butter together in a double boiler, and warm on very low heat, just enough to thoroughly warm. Add in the beeswax or carnauba wax pastilles and gently whisk until they've completely dissolved into the oil mixture. Next, pour the hydrosol, vitamin E, and essential oils into your blender. Turn the blender on low and slowly add the warmed oil mixture into the center of the blender in a slow, steady stream. It all has to be mixed together completely to ensure that the hand cream emulsifies properly and doesn't clump up. Use your spatula to scrape the edges. This will scoop up any unmixed bits and ensure a creamy texture. Once you've done this, turn the blender on low to finish mixing the cream.

Use a spatula to scrape the cream out of the blender and use a spoon to decant into the empty jars. Lid and label the jars with a date and the essential oils that you used. Keep the extra jars in the refrigerator to last longer. This cream can last 6 to 10 months stored in the refrigerator. Always smell it or look for mold to ensure it's still fresh.

LAVENDER AND HONEY BODY WASH

This is a small batch recipe; feel free to double it to save time. Lavender essential oil and honey are soothing for many skin types. Lavender is known as the calming essential oil and is ideal for keeping skin soft and nourished. Use 10 drops of lavender for children six years old and younger.

YIELD: 10-ounce pump dispenser

1 cup unscented baby mild Castile soap

⅓ cup organic honey

1 tablespoon fractionated coconut oil

1 teaspoon vitamin E

3 teaspoons vegetable glycerin

25 drops lavender

DIRECTIONS: In a mixing bowl, whisk together all of the ingredients until completely blended. Transfer body soap mixture into a plastic pump bottle. Apply 2 to 3 pumps for each shower.

NOURISHING FACIAL MASK

Facial masks nourish and cleanse your skin. Bentonite and green French clay bind to toxins and skin impurities and gently remove them, revealing fresh, healthy skin. Helichrysum, frankincense, and geranium are great for antiaging properties and skin rejuvenation. These essential oils can reduce the appearance of fine lines and wrinkles, leaving your skin smoother after application.

This mask is designed for all skin types and is safe to use once a week to achieve best results. You can find bentonite clay at your local health food store. Make sure to avoid metal spoons and bowls when using the clay.

YIELD: 1 application

2½ teaspoons bentonite clay or green French clay

2 teaspoons apply cider vinegar

1 drop helichrysum essential oil

1 drop frankincense essential oil

1 drop geranium essential oil

DIRECTIONS: Combine bentonite clay and vinegar in a small plastic bowl and stir until completely combined. Add essential oils to the clay mixture. Apply with fingertips around the face and neck, avoiding the eyes and mouth. Let the mask dry for 10 to 20 minutes. Rinse with warm water and follow it up with the Homemade Citrus Body Butter recipe on page 123.

WHITENING/REMINERALIZING TOOTHPASTE

YIELD: 4-ounce tube or glass jar

5 tablespoons calcium carbonate

3 tablespoons xylitol

4 tablespoons raw organic coconut oil

2 to 3 tablespoons distilled water

2 tablespoons bentonite clay

20 to 30 drops essential oil (this seems like a lot, but the clay soaks it up)

DIRECTIONS: Mix all ingredients but clay and EOs in a food processor (you can do it by hand, but the food processor is faster and more efficient). Slowly add clay with a plastic spoon or silicon spatula and mix until smooth. A kid's plastic fork works great for mushing it. Add desired amount of EOs and mix. Store in a silicone squeeze tube, which is a more sanitary option, or a glass jar.

Note: Do not use metal with the clay, as metal will deactivate it. Travel-size silicone GoToob tubes are great for this recipe and the other toothpaste recipes to follow.

OPTIONAL FLAVORS:

30 drops peppermint essential oil

15 drops spearmint and 15 drops peppermint essential oil

20 drops wild orange and 10 drops peppermint/spearmint essential oil

30 drops wild orange for children under age 12

TEETH-WHITENING PASTE

YIELD: 4-ounce tube or glass jar

⅔ cup baking soda

2 tablespoons hydrogen peroxide

2 tablespoons fractionated or melted coconut oil

6 drops peppermint essential oil

Filtered water as needed for consistency

DIRECTIONS: Mix all ingredients in a small bowl with a spoon. Slowly stir in filtered water until you reach a consistent paste. Mix well so that the paste is not clumpy. To use, apply the whitening paste to your toothbrush and brush for 3 to 4 minutes. This allows time for your teeth to whiten. Apply 3 to 4 times a week for 4 weeks for optimal results.

MINTY NATURAL TOOTHPASTE

This toothpaste recipe is designed for sensitive teeth. Peppermint, clove, and cinnamon essential oils are ideal for oral and gum health. Clove essential oil is a powerful antioxidant and has been used by dentists for its oral repair properties. Peppermint and cinnamon keep the mouth clean and kissable.

YIELD: 4-ounce tube or glass jar

⅔ cup baking soda

1 teaspoon sea salt

½ teaspoon organic stevia powder

2 tablespoons fractionated or melted coconut oil

5 drops peppermint essential oil

2 drops clove essential oil

2 drops cinnamon essential oil

Filtered water as needed for consistency

DIRECTIONS: Mix all ingredients in a small bowl with a spoon. Slowly stir in filtered water until you reach the consistency of toothpaste. Mix well so that the paste is not clumpy. Apply a small amount to your toothbrush when brushing your teeth.

CHAPTER

❖7❖

AROMATHERAPY BLENDS FOR MOOD, FOCUS, AND PURIFYING

Your sense of smell is directly connected to the way you experience the world around you. Aroma has a way of elevating your experiences and connecting to your memory and emotions. Imagine walking into your grandma's kitchen during the holidays and smelling her famous apple cider with clove, cinnamon, and other spices. That aromatic combination triggers nostalgic feelings and joyful memories of growing up. When I open a bottle of wild orange essential oil, I am always taken back to the orange groves near my family's home. Wild orange elicits feelings of happiness, calm, and abundance each time I open the bottle and take a direct inhalation. Of the five senses, the sense of smell is the most powerful and influential due to its direct connection to the limbic brain. Your sense of smell can detect thousands of odor varieties and elicit infinitesimal emotional responses. Recent research has discovered that the sense of smell is directly link to emotional, mental, and physical well-being.

The Power of Essential Oil Aromatherapy

One of the most researched areas of aromatherapy is the effect essential oils have on emotions and mood. The moment you open a bottle of essential oils, you will immediately experience the aroma of that single essential oil or blend of essential oils. As defined, essential oils are volatile aromatic compounds rich in complexity. Due to their volatile nature, aroma is an intrinsic part of essential oils. In a chemical sense, aroma is the interaction of individual chemical constituents (in this case, essential oil constituents) that interact with olfactory receptors in the nose. These olfactory receptors then carry these chemical messages to the emotional and memory center of the brain. The chemistry of essential oils differs greatly, which explains why essential oils make up many different aromas that can affect us in many ways, especially when it comes to mood.

How Aroma Influences Us

Scent is an amazingly powerful tool that can be used to influence your well-being in a multitude of ways. Since the 1990s, there has been convincing research demonstrating that simply breathing an essential oil aroma is effective for calming anxious feelings in multiple environmental settings. The olfactory receptors located in the upper nasal cavity make direct connections with the limbic system of the brain, an area of the brain that regulates the body's emotional responses. This intrinsic connection between aroma and emotion becomes obvious in daily life as certain aromas trigger memories or specific feelings. Some odors directly impact mood (e.g., they can be calming, energizing, or motivating), while others trigger specific memories that are tied to a specific, strong emotion. Due to the direct link of the olfactory system to this area of the brain, aroma is capable of interacting directly with the hypothalamus, influencing neurochemistry throughout the body, and, in turn, potentiating powerful health outcomes.

Smart moms understand the implications of emotion on overall well-being for themselves and their family. There are many acceptable ways to use essential oils for their aromatic properties. One method is to diffuse the oil into the air, as I mentioned in Chapter 2. Not only does diffusion make the oil accessible to the body, but research indicates that there are air purification benefits when diffusing oils.

When diffusing essential oils, an ultrasonic cool-air diffuser or cool-air nebulizing diffuser is best because burning or heating essential oils can alter their delicate chemistry. If a diffuser is not available, simply dropping essential oils into the palm of the hand and then cupping around the nose and breathing deeply is a convenient method for using essential oils at any time, in any situation. I personally breathe in essential oils by cupping my hand several times a day. Although there are many ways that essential oils can be applied, throughout my experience as a practitioner I have found that repeated daily exposure to the aroma of essential oils provides unique and significant support to healthy function of the body and mind.

In this chapter I am going to share with you many powerful aromatherapy blends that I have tested over the years. These blends are designed to support emotions and mood along with focus and concentration. I will also share favorite blends designed to purify the air in your home or office and provide a healthy environment for the family or workplace. Many of the blends featured in this chapter are designed for diffusers, but many of them can also be used topically when diluted according to the chart on page 36.

You can also pre-make these blends and have them ready for direct inhalation, right out of the bottle. The two best ways for direct inhalation are either taking deep breaths from the bottle or applying a couple of drops to your palms, rubbing them together, and taking three to four deep breaths.

When diffusing in an ultrasonic cool-air diffuser, I recommend using five to eight drops of a single essential oil or essential oil blend, such as the blends found in this chapter. When using a cool-air nebulizing diffuser, the essential oil bottle is typically attached directly to the diffuser. For the cool-air nebulizing diffuser, I recommend premixing the blends at a 10x concentration in a 10- to 15-milliliter essential oil bottle to ensure you have enough essential oil to run the diffuser. It's worth noting that diffusers differ in size and type, so feel free to experiment with the amount of essential oil drops you use in your personal ultrasonic cool-air diffuser or cool-air nebulizing diffuser.

I want to encourage you to have fun with aromatherapy blends. Come up with new combinations for your own home, especially for different seasons and depending on the mood you want to elicit in the house.

Calming Blends

SLEEPY-TIME DIFFUSER BLEND

This blend is ideal to unwind for a restful night's sleep. Lavender and vetiver are an excellent combination for calming the mind. Roman chamomile is known as the peacekeeper essential oil and blends beautifully with lavender and vetiver.

Consider diffusing this blend right before bed and continue to run it after you fall asleep for a peaceful slumber.

YIELD: 1 application

2 drops lavender essential oil

1 drop vetiver essential oil

1 drop Roman chamomile essential oil

DIRECTIONS: Add essential oil to an ultrasonic cool-air diffuser. If using a cool-air nebulizing diffuser, multiply this blend by 10 in a 15-milliliter glass bottle and run for 30 minutes to 1 hour before going to bed.

GOODNIGHT MENTAL CHATTER

Shutting off the brain can be challenging at night, especially with the numerous uncompleted tasks and checklists in your head. This blend is effective at helping to shut off the mental chatter and get a restful night's sleep.

Bergamot is known as the essential oil of self-love. This essential oil combined with lavender and clary sage sets the tone for a calming mood.

YIELD: 1 application

2 drops clary sage essential oil

2 drop lavender essential oil

1 drop bergamot essential oil

DIRECTIONS: Add essential oils to an ultrasonic cool-air diffuser. If using a cool-air nebulizing diffuser, multiply this blend by 10 in a 15-milliliter glass bottle and run for 30 minutes to 1 hour before going to bed.

SUNDAY SNUGGLE BLEND

Create a family snuggle session any day of the week with this fun blend. Vetiver and juniper berry promote a calming environment. Bergamot essential oil is known as the self-love oil and promotes connection.

YIELD: 1 application

3 drops bergamot essential oil

2 drops vetiver essential oil

1 drop juniper berry essential oil

DIRECTIONS: Add essential oils to an ultrasonic cool-air diffuser. If using a cool-air nebulizing diffuser, multiply this blend by 10 in a 15-milliliter glass bottle and run for 30 minutes to 1 hour, or apply 1 to 2 drops of blend to palms and take 3 to 5 deep belly breaths.

SELF-LOVE BLEND

Bergamot is known as the "self-love" and "self-acceptance" essential oil. This blend is rich and beautiful and will get you back to that place of honoring the self.

YIELD: 1 application

3 drops bergamot essential oil

2 drops cedarwood essential oil

1 drop jasmine essential oil

DIRECTIONS: Add essential oils to an ultrasonic cool-air diffuser. If using a cool-air nebulizing diffuser, multiply this blend by 10 in a 15-milliliter glass bottle and run for 30 minutes to 1 hour, or apply 1 to 2 drops of blend to palms and take 3 to 5 deep belly breaths.

CALMING MEDITATION BLEND

Frankincense and cedarwood have been historically used in meditation practice to quiet the mind. Wild orange balances out the frankincense and cedarwood with a pleasant citrus aroma, and rosemary promotes focus and concentration.

YIELD: 1 application

2 drops frankincense essential oil

2 drops cedarwood essential oil

2 drops wild orange essential oil

1 drop rosemary essential oil

DIRECTIONS: Add essential oils to an ultrasonic cool-air diffuser. If using a cool-air nebulizing diffuser, multiply this blend by 10 in a 15-milliliter glass bottle and run for 30 minutes to 1 hour, or apply 1 to 2 drops of blend to palms and take 3 to 5 deep belly breaths.

Mood Balance Blends

ABUNDANCE BLEND

This is my favorite abundance blend to set the tone for my day when I am writing in my gratitude journal in the mornings. Learn more about this powerful morning ritual on page 160.

YIELD: 1 application

2 drops frankincense

2 drops wild orange

1 drop peppermint

DIRECTIONS: Add essential oils to an ultrasonic cool-air diffuser. If using a cool-air nebulizing diffuser, multiply this blend by 10 in a 15-milliliter glass bottle and run for 30 minutes to 1 hour. Or, achieve an instant sense of abundance by applying 1 drop of each oil to your palms, rubbing your palms together, and breathing in the aroma with 3 to 5 deep belly breaths.

MOTIVATION BLEND

This is my favorite blend for getting my morning started with energy and motivation.

YIELD: 1 application

3 drops sandalwood essential oil

3 drops bergamot essential oil

2 drops ginger essential oil

1 drop lime essential oil

DIRECTIONS: Add essential oils to an ultrasonic cool-air diffuser. If using a cool-air nebulizing diffuser, multiply this blend by 10 in a 15-milliliter glass bottle and run for 30 minutes to 1 hour, or apply 1 to 2 drops of blend to palms and take 3 to 5 deep belly breaths.

LET IT GO EMOTIONAL RELEASE BLEND

When built-up emotions are creating sad feelings, this blend acts as emotional cleanser.

YIELD: 1 application

3 drops tangerine essential oil

2 drops bergamot essential oil

1 drop jasmine essential oil

1 drop ylang ylang essential oil

DIRECTIONS: Add essential oils to an ultrasonic cool-air diffuser. If using a cool-air nebulizing diffuser, multiply this blend by 10 in a 15-milliliter glass bottle and run for 30 minutes to 1 hour, or apply 1 to 2 drops of blend to palms and take 3 to 5 deep belly breaths for instant mood calming.

CALM THE BEAST BLEND

Sandalwood, lavender, and clary sage are effective at calming and centering the mind during moments of anxiousness or irritation. Vanilla aids to enhance your mood.

YIELD: 1 application

2 drops clary sage essential oil

2 drops lavender essential oil

1 drop sandalwood essential oil

1 drop vanilla essential oil

DIRECTIONS: Add essential oils to an ultrasonic cool-air diffuser. If using a cool-air nebulizing diffuser, multiply this blend by 10 in a 15-milliliter glass bottle and run for 30 minutes to 1 hour, or apply 1 to 2 drops to palms and take 3 to 5 deep belly breaths for instant mood balance.

ANXIOUS FEELINGS BLEND

Anxious feelings can arise out of nowhere. This blend calms the mind and relaxes the senses so that the anxious feeling moves through you. Take 3 to 5 deep belly breaths for immediate support.

YIELD: 1 application

2 drops cedarwood essential oil

2 drops wild orange essential oil

1 drop ylang ylang essential oil

1 drop patchouli essential oil

DIRECTIONS: Add essential oils to an ultrasonic cool-air diffuser. If using a cool-air nebulizing diffuser, multiply this blend by 10 in a 15-milliter glass bottle and run for 30 minutes to 1 hour.

NEGATIVE SELF-TALK SUPPORT BLEND

This blend helps to stop negative self-talk patterns that arise. Wild orange and bergamot citrus oil help release negative emotions and promote happy thoughts. Clary sage is known for counteracting sad feelings and creating emotional ease.

YIELD: 1 application

3 drops bergamot essential oil

2 drops clary sage essential oil

1 drop wild orange essential oil

DIRECTIONS: Add essential oils to an ultrasonic cool-air diffuser. If using a cool-air nebulizing diffuser, multiply this blend by 10 in a 15-milliliter glass bottle and run for 30 minutes to 1 hour, or apply 1 to 2 drops of the blend to palms and take 3 to 5 deep belly breaths to quiet the self-talk. You can also apply this blend topically to pulse points on the wrist, behind the ears, and temples. Make sure to dilute accordingly when applying topically.

OVERWHELM RESET BLEND

This blend supports the mind in letting go of overwhelm after dealing with a hectic day, and is also very effective as a rollerball bottle blend. Simply add 30 drops of the blend to a 10-milliliter rollerball bottle and fill the rest up with almond oil. Roll onto wrists, feet, temples, and back of neck.

YIELD: 1 application

2 drops geranium essential oil

2 drops clary sage essential oil

1 drop patchouli essential oil

1 drop ylang ylang essential oil

DIRECTIONS: Add essential oils to an ultrasonic cool-air diffuser. If using a cool-air nebulizing diffuser, multiply this blend by 10 in a 15-milliliter glass bottle and run for 30 minutes to 1 hour, or apply 1 to 2 drops of the blend to palms and take 3 to 5 deep belly breaths.

Focus Blends

BRAIN FOG BUSTER BLEND

Lemon, peppermint, and rosemary create a synergistic blend that will support memory and concentration, and provide an energy boost to help with moments of brain fog.

YIELD: 1 application

2 drops lemon essential oil

2 drop peppermint essential oil

1 drop rosemary essential oil

DIRECTIONS: Add essential oils to an ultrasonic cool-air diffuser. If using a cool-air nebulizing diffuser, multiply this blend by 10 in a 15-milliliter glass bottle and run for 30 minutes to 1 hour, or apply 1 to 2 drops of the blend to palms and take 3 to 5 deep belly breaths. You can also apply this blend topically to pulse points on the wrist, behind the ears, and on the neck. Make sure to dilute accordingly when applying topically.

MENTAL CLARITY BLEND

Get ready for your brain to feel more clear and sharp when processing information or working on a big project. Juniper berry and rosemary are known to support brain function and awaken the senses. Peppermint and grapefruit are ideal for invigorating and inspiring you to gain clarity.

YIELD: 1 application

3 drops grapefruit essential oil

2 drops juniper berry essential oil

1 drop rosemary essential oil

1 drop peppermint essential oil

DIRECTIONS: Add essential oils to an ultrasonic cool-air diffuser. If using a cool-air nebulizing diffuser, multiply this blend by 10 in a 15-milliliter glass bottle and run for 30 minutes to 1 hour, or apply 1 to 2 drops of the blend to palms and take 3 to 5 deep belly breaths.

FOCUS AND CONCENTRATION BLEND

This blend is ideal for stimulating focus and concentration during long tasks and homework. Rosemary is known as a powerful memory-boosting oil. Grapefruit and ylang ylang are a perfect duo for invigoration and motivation.

YIELD: 1 application

2 drops grapefruit essential oil

2 drops rosemary essential oil

1 drop ylang ylang essential oil

DIRECTIONS: Add essential oils to an ultrasonic cool-air diffuser. If using a cool-air nebulizing diffuser, multiply this blend by 10 in a 15-milliliter glass bottle and run for 30 minutes to 1 hour.

Energizing and Uplifting Blends

MORNING WAKE-UP BLEND

One of my favorite ways to start each morning is with this wake-up blend. The blend of peppermint and citrus is invigorating, and they awaken the senses instantly to help you start your day on the right foot. A drop of ylang ylang balances the aroma and makes for a pleasant and effective morning routine.

YIELD: 1 application

2 drops wild orange essential oil

2 drops peppermint essential oil

1 drop ylang ylang essential oil

DIRECTIONS: Add essential oils to an ultrasonic cool-air diffuser. If using a cool-air nebulizing diffuser, multiply this blend by 10 in a 15-milliliter glass bottle and run for 30 minutes to 1 hour, or apply 1 to 2 drops of the blend to palms and take 3 to 5 deep belly breaths.

FIGHT FATIGUE BLEND

Say goodbye to that mid-afternoon slump. This blend is equally beneficial for kids when using the spearmint essential oil.

YIELD: 1 application

5 drops bergamot essential oil

3 drops grapefruit essential oil

2 drops peppermint or spearmint essential oil

DIRECTIONS: Add essential oils to an ultrasonic cool-air diffuser. If using a cool-air nebulizing diffuser, multiply this blend by 10 in a 15-milliliter glass bottle and run for 30 minutes to 1 hour, or apply 1 to 2 drops of the blend to palms and take 3 to 5 deep belly breaths.

LIQUID SUNSHINE BLEND

Sunshine comes to the rescue during those days when sad feelings are surfacing. This blend is effective at promoting happy feelings.

YIELD: 1 application

3 drops grapefruit essential oil

2 drops tangerine essential oil

1 drop spearmint essential oil

DIRECTIONS: Add essential oils to an ultrasonic cool-air diffuser. If using a cool-air nebulizing diffuser, multiply this blend by 10 in a 15-milliliter glass bottle and run for 30 minutes to 1 hour, or apply 1 to 2 drops of the blend to palms and take 3 to 5 deep belly breaths.

INSTANT ENERGY BLEND

This is my favorite energizer blend for a quick pick-me-up, especially when working on a big project or juggling multiple tasks at once.

YIELD: 1 application

1 drop wild orange essential oil

1 drop peppermint essential oil

DIRECTIONS: Achieve an instant energy boost by applying the essential oils to your palms. Rub your palms together and breathe in the aroma of the essential oil blend with 3 to 5 deep belly breaths.

TROPICAL ESCAPE BLEND

This blend always reminds me of relaxing on the beach on a tropical island. When you need a quick escape, try diffusing this blend while looking at photos of your favorite island vacation.

YIELD: 1 application

3 drops tangerine essential oil

3 drops grapefruit essential oil

2 drops sandalwood essential oil

DIRECTIONS: Add essential oils to an ultrasonic cool-air diffuser. If using a cool-air nebulizing diffuser, multiply this blend by 10 in a 15-milliliter glass bottle and run for 30 minutes to 1 hour. Or, apply to palms and take 3 to 5 deep belly breaths.

VITALITY BLEND

For those days that you need to feel revitalized, this is the perfect blend for you. Citrus and mint energize you, and frankincense promotes positive and uplifting feelings.

YIELD: 1 application

3 drops lemon essential oil

3 drops wild orange essential oil

2 drops peppermint essential oil

1 drop frankincense essential oil

DIRECTIONS: Add essential oils to an ultrasonic cool-air diffuser. If using a cool-air nebulizing diffuser, multiply this blend by 10 in a 15-milliliter glass bottle and run for 30 minutes to 1 hour, or apply to palms and take 3 to 5 deep belly breaths for instant mood-lifting support.

Air-Purifying Blends

MAN CAVE BLEND

Even men need some aromatic mood support. This blend not only freshens the air in a man cave, it's a great blend to support motivation and concentration for any tasks in the "cave."

YIELD: 1 application

3 drops lime essential oil

2 drops vetiver essential oil

1 drop patchouli essential oil

DIRECTIONS: Add essential oils to an ultrasonic cool-air diffuser. If using a cool-air nebulizing diffuser, multiply this blend by 10 in a 15-milliliter glass bottle and run for 30 minutes to 1 hour, or apply 1 to 2 drops of the blend to palms and take 3 to 5 deep belly breaths.

CLEAN KITCHEN BLEND

All four of these essential oils are incredible for supporting a healthy immune system, uplifting mood, and purifying the air in the home. This blend is perfect for the kitchen, bathroom, and areas of the home that need a fresh scent.

YIELD: 1 application

3 drops lime essential oil

2 drops lemon essential oil

2 drops lavender essential oil

2 drops rosemary essential oil

DIRECTIONS: Add essential oils to an ultrasonic cool-air diffuser. If using a cool-air nebulizing diffuser, multiply this blend by 10 in a 15-milliliter glass bottle and run for 30 minutes to 1 hour.

CITRUS ODOR ELIMINATION BLEND

This blend is the perfect solution any time you need to eliminate odor in your home. Citrus essential oils are clean and purifying, and also create harmony in your home. Adding one drop of basil creates an invigorating and clean scent when combined with lime and bergamot.

YIELD: 1 application

2 drops bergamot essential oil

2 drops lime essential oil

1 drop basil essential oil

1 drop lemon essential oil

DIRECTIONS: Add essential oils to an ultrasonic cool-air diffuser. If using a cool-air nebulizing diffuser, multiply this blend by 10 in a 15-milliliter glass bottle and run for 30 minutes to 1 hour.

FLORAL SURPRISE BLEND

This blend is the perfect garden scent, ideal for the weekends or during springtime. This blend also contains some of the most effective female support essential oils.

YIELD: 1 application

2 drops lavender essential oil

2 drops clary sage essential oil

2 drops geranium essential oil

1 drop ylang ylang essential oil

DIRECTIONS: Add essential oils to an ultrasonic cool-air diffuser. If using a cool-air nebulizing diffuser, multiply this blend by 10 in a 15-milliliter glass bottle and run for 30 minutes to 1 hour.

BREATHE DEEP BLEND

Use this blend of oils for respiratory support, especially during bedtime. This blend will help open up airways for a restful night's sleep.

YIELD: 1 application

2 drops cardamom essential oil

1 drop lemon essential oil

1 drop lime essential oil

1 drop rosemary essential oil

DIRECTIONS: Add essential oils to an ultrasonic cool-air diffuser. If using a cool-air nebulizing diffuser, multiply this blend by 10 in a 15-milliliter glass bottle and run for 30 minutes to 1 hour, or apply 1 to 2 drops of the blend to palms and take 3 to 5 deep belly breaths.

WALK IN THE FOREST BLEND

This is another incredible meditation or recharge blend. I love to blend this in the morning, enjoying it with a cup of tea and my journal.

YIELD: 1 application

1 drop frankincense essential oil

1 drop juniper berry essential oil

1 drop eucalyptus essential oil

3 drops grapefruit essential oil

DIRECTIONS: Add essential oils to an ultrasonic cool-air diffuser. If using a cool-air nebulizing diffuser, multiply this blend by 10 in a 15-milliliter glass bottle and run for 30 minutes to 1 hour.

COZY AUTUMN BLEND

This is my favorite fall seasonal blend for nighttime, when everyone is winding down and relaxing.

YIELD: 1 application

3 drops tangerine essential oil

1 drop ginger essential oil

1 drop clove essential oil

1 drop frankincense essential oil

DIRECTIONS: Add essential oils to an ultrasonic cool-air diffuser. If using a cool-air nebulizing diffuser, multiply this blend by 10 in a 15-milliliter glass bottle and run for 30 minutes to 1 hour.

CHAPTER

SELF-CARE WELLNESS RITUALS WITH ESSENTIAL OILS

Do you ever forget to take care of yourself?

When it comes to being a mom, I have a feeling the answer is *yes*. When you stop prioritizing self-care, everything else follows suit—your confidence is depleted; your energy is zapped; you may be operating in a mental fog where it's hard to care about anything or anyone. You may experience feeling rundown and even apathetic.

Self-care is an important part of your wellness routine, and it often goes by the wayside in this overscheduled, hyper-connected world. Consumed by "being busy," we often forget to take time for ourselves and take care of our bodies. We tend to place other people's needs before our own healthcare needs and suffer the health consequences over time.

These consequences wreak havoc on your mood, energy, sleep, weight, and overall quality of life.

Practicing self-care rituals creates mindfulness and brings balance into your life. You'll feel more connected to yourself and the world around you. Rituals are designed to help you celebrate moments of magic wherever you are. Every aspect of life is punctuated with ritual. To indulge in self-care is to connect with nature, surround yourself with beauty, thrive in your community, and experiment with new healthy lifestyle practices that enhance the quality of your life and the lives of those around you. When you attune to what I call the magic of being present, wherever you may be, gratitude allows you to honor each moment as sacred and show up with energy and grace.

When establishing self-care rituals, essential oils can act as a bridge for maintaining and supporting daily, weekly, and monthly habits. Essential oils allow for you to indulge your senses and deepen your moments of relaxation and rejuvenation. They act as adaptogens to support mood, hormones, the immune system, and overall homeostasis. They can be calming and energizing while supporting your body on a cellular level. In this guide, I will share my favorite recipes and natural solutions to enhance your self-care rituals.

These rituals are designed to reinforce healthy habits and beliefs to nourish your body, mind, and soul. My recommendation is to pick one to three rituals that really resonate with you and schedule them into your daily and weekly calendar, especially if you feel your life is too busy. After several weeks of practicing these self-care rituals, you will have more energy and abundance to show up even bigger for your family and community, and most importantly, *you*!

I want to encourage you to start with your morning routine. Morning rituals are the most important for creating powerful healthy habits for you and the entire family. Morning rituals lay the groundwork for the life that you want to create each and every day. Now, let's create it!

Morning Rituals: Set the Tone for Your Day

"How you start your day is often how you live your life." —Louise Hay

Your morning self-care routine is all about setting the tone for your day. Each day, we get to choose the day that we are going to have, and morning rituals really allow that to come into reality. This is when you have your opportunity to choose your intention and flow for the day. Not every day is the same. If you wake without a morning routine, you will be subjected to a random flow that depends on other people's needs and agendas, your caffeine intake, and your blood sugar levels. Set your body and mind for success in the morning with rituals that will support you throughout the day, especially when you have a lot on your plate. Here are some powerful rituals to consider for the beginning of the day. This may mean getting up a half hour earlier to have this time to yourself, but I promise you, it's worth it.

Gratitude Journaling

Taking a moment to write down what you are grateful for in life is arguably one of the most important steps of your morning routine, in my opinion. This is something that I have been doing for years and can't imagine starting my day without. This step is about personal growth, making positive daily change, and contributing to your self-care first thing in the morning. And it only takes 5 to 10 minutes. All you need is a notebook or journal, a pen, and my favorite essential oil blend: Gratitude Blend. This blend awakens the mind and allows you to hack into your happy chemicals to get you centered to start your day.

GRATITUDE BLEND

YIELD: 1 application

2 drops frankincense essential oil

2 drops bergamot essential oil

1 drop ylang ylang essential oil

DIRECTIONS: Before beginning your gratitude journal or meditation ritual, add the blend to your hands, rub your hands together, and take 3 deep belly breaths with this blend. You can substitute sandalwood for frankincense if you prefer. Other essential blends to consider are Focus and Concentration Blend (page 151), Self-Love Blend (page 146), and Motivation Blend (page 147).

Establish a Meditation Practice

When it comes to a meditation practice, you only need a few minutes. There is no wrong way to meditate and no set amount of time. I recommend five minutes for meditation. Your meditation ritual may vary day to day, depending on your needs. Meditation allows you to gain mental clarity and set an intention for your best day.

Set up a sacred space in your home where you can sit in silence and turn inward. Deep breathing and focused concentration slows down brain waves, making them more organized. It allows you to activate the parasympathetic nervous system, releasing endorphins in the bloodstream and allowing the brain to emit happy hormones. This helps you have presence and peace of mind, and maintain a practice of gratitude.

Use the Calming Meditation Blend or even just wild orange to start your meditation practice for brain-boosting benefits. If you prefer sandalwood essential oil for meditation, feel free to substitute it for frankincense. Sesquiterpenes, found in cedarwood, myrrh, frankincense, and vetiver, are ideal for mental clarity and focus.

CALMING MEDITATION BLEND

YIELD: 1 application

1 drop frankincense essential oil

1 drop cedarwood essential oil

1 drop wild orange essential oil

1 drop rosemary essential oil

DIRECTIONS: Apply 1 drop of each essential oil into your palms. Rub your palms together and take 3 to 5 deep belly breaths before starting your meditation. Apply the remaining essential oil to your palms and on the back of your neck for added benefit.

Exercise and Yoga

Motion is life, and moving your body in the morning is great for feeling energized, loving your heart, and getting focused on the tasks for the day. A 10- to 15-minute brisk walk or 5 to 10 minutes of yoga in your living room is exactly what the doctor ordered. Taking a whiff of peppermint and grapefruit essential oil will help energize your mind and body. Try the Instant Energy Blend (page 153) or Vitality Blend (page 154) prior to moving your body.

My favorite morning yoga practice starts with the sun salutation sequence. Practicing at least three sun salutations in the morning is a wonderful way to awaken your body, stretch, and say good morning to all of your muscles. The sun salutation is also a great way to know your body and its limits, since in the morning you are "raw," so to speak—your muscles and joints still need to be warmed up. Practice being gentle with yourself.

Feel free to practice your morning sun salutations with modifications depending on the needs of your body. This will set you up for success the rest of the day.

Get Hydrated

Make drinking water a priority every morning. If you forget to start your day with an adequate water intake, you are likely to remain dehydrated for the rest of the day and feel tired and sluggish. Hydrating your body and cells with 16 to 32 ounces of water first thing in the morning is one of the best rituals you can implement for yourself and it only takes a couple minutes.

Drinking water first thing in the morning helps with mental clarity, energy, mood, and skin complexion. When you hydrate first thing in the morning, you replenish fluids lost from sweating and urinating throughout the evening, and provide the water your cells need to function properly.

If you don't enjoy the taste of water or you are looking for ways to incorporate antioxidants into your water, I recommend making a water infusion two to three times a week. Dressing up your water with an infusion of herbs, essential oils, and/or fruits is a great way to drink delicious water throughout the day. I have included one of my favorite recipes from my *Water Infusions* book below. I love to start my day with this recipe because you can find the ingredients all year long and it's incredibly renewing. If you would like more water infusion ideas, please check out *Water Infusions* for recipes on detox, energy, and renewal.

DETOX AND RENEW WATER INFUSION

YIELD: 1 pitcher

½ cup blueberries

1 lemon, sliced

½ cup sliced cucumber

1½ liters water

2 drops lemon essential oil

DIRECTIONS: In a small bowl, muddle blueberries. Combine muddled blueberries, lemon, and cucumber slices into a 2-quart pitcher along with the water. Add lemon oil and stir. Refrigerate for 3 to 5 hours before serving. May be consumed at room temperature, or chilled with ice. Keep refrigerated and consume within 2 to 3 days.

Morning Green Smoothie

Drinking green smoothies every day is one of the easiest and best habits you can have if you want to see an improvement in your energy levels. Drinking your green smoothie for breakfast is also a great way to start the day. It only takes a few minutes to prepare. This is my absolute best daily habit/tip that will increase your nutritional intake by 700 percent. I take my green smoothie on the go each morning or sip on it as I start my morning routine. Fueling your body in the morning is the best way to set yourself up for success.

Now if that is not convincing enough, a daily green smoothie can also increase your fiber intake, ramp up your fruit and vegetable intake, and of course, support your energy levels.

POPEYE GOES TO THAILAND GREEN SMOOTHIE

This is just one way to use essential oils in green smoothie recipes. Play around with your favorite fruits and vegetables to create a delicious and energy-boosting smoothie that nourishes your body, fights fatigue, and tastes amazing at the same time! For more green smoothie recipes, check out my other book, *The DASH Diet Cookbook*.

YIELD: 1 smoothie

3 handfuls spinach

1 cup frozen or fresh mango

15 mint leaves

½ cup frozen or fresh strawberries

½ banana

2 cups coconut water or filtered water

2 drops lemon or wild orange essential oil

DIRECTIONS: Place all of the ingredients in a high-speed blender, and blend until smooth.

Note: Blend spinach and coconut water by themselves first for the smoothest consistency.

Two-Minute Shower Ritual

We all shower sometime during the day to clean our bodies. If you typically take a morning shower to wake up and feel refreshed, here is a great ritual for you. Each morning when you take a hot, steamy shower, add this essential oil blend into your palm and breathe in. This 2-minute ritual will open your airways, send oxygen to the body and brain, awaken your senses, and energize you. Before getting in the shower, grab one to three essential oils or a blend that really resonates with you that day. I recommend keeping the Mental Clarity Blend (page 151) or Breathe Deep Blend (page 156) in your shower or trying out these invigorating oils: grapefruit, wild orange, peppermint, and eucalyptus. Below is my favorite shower blend to use for your next shower. It reminds me of living on the coast.

COASTAL LIVING SHOWER BLEND

YIELD: 1 application

2 drops frankincense essential oil

2 drops cedarwood essential oil

1 drop rosemary essential oil

2 drops wild orange essential oil

DIRECTIONS: In the hot shower, add two to three drops of this essential oil blend into your palm and breathe in.

Adorn Your Way to a Good Mood

"There is a science (enclothed cognition) about how what you wear influences the way you feel. Reframe 'getting dressed' in the morning to 'adorning yourself,' and the moments you spend preparing yourself for the day are charged with ritual." —Latham Thomas

Just because it's gloomy outside doesn't mean you need to reflect that in the way that you dress yourself. I like to take this ritual a step further and adorn myself throughout the day with mood-boosting essential oils. To be honest, I don't always adorn myself with the best clothing; sometimes I live in yoga pants from morning till I go to bed, but I do use essential oils all day long, especially for mood balance and energy.

For your morning "adorning ritual," choose a blend of oils that will support your mood for the day. I love adorning myself with essential oils that make me feel abundant and energized. Be your own alchemist and choose a blend that resonates with your mood and abundance mindset. Essential oils that are wonderful to combine are clary sage, bergamot, jasmine, sandalwood, and ylang ylang. Below is a beautiful superwoman rollerball bottle blend for inspiring your inner rock star!

SUPERWOMAN BLEND

YIELD: 10-milliliter rollerball bottle

12 drops sandalwood essential oil

10 drops clary sage essential oil

8 drops bergamot essential oil

4 drop ylang ylang essential oil

fractionated coconut oil or almond oil

DIRECTIONS: Place the essential oil in a 10-milliliter rollerball bottle and then fill to the top with your carrier oil of choice. Roll the blends over the pulse points on your neck, ankles, and wrists.

Evening Routine

"Rest and self-care are so important. When you take time to replenish your spirit, it allows you to serve others from the overflow. You cannot serve from an empty vessel." -Eleanor Brown

I am an advocate for evening rituals in order to de-stress and get centered after the busyness of the day. Equally important to starting your day with morning rituals that fuel your mind and body, evening rituals are critical to replenishing your cup from all that you gave during the day.

I know that a lot of moms would say that they don't have time for an evening routine. Many moms want to get things done while their children are sleeping. Although accomplishing tasks are important, replenishing your energy is equally necessary. I want to encourage you to create 10 to 30 minutes in the evening to focus on relaxing and preparing for a restful night's sleep. In this section I have chosen rituals that are indulgent and relaxing. Some of the evening rituals are 30 minutes long and others only take a couple minutes to implement. Choose one or two rituals that you can commit to each night, and experience a sense of renewal that accompanies a restful night's sleep.

Therapeutic Bath

The sea is nature's medicine. Preparing a therapeutic sea salt bath helps to support clearing out toxins from your body and can cleanse and ground you when you feel spaced out, overwhelmed, or not at home in your own skin. During your bath, consider taking deep belly breaths with lavender or clary sage essential oil. Imagine that each breath is releasing all of the daily stressors. To help ease tension, take a moment to stretch your neck and shoulder muscles, and stretch your back by reaching for your toes.

BATH SOAK RECIPE

This is my favorite recipe for a quick and relaxing bath soak. Another option for a bath soak is the Chamomile Lavender Oatmeal Milk Bath, found on page 122. Feel free to choose two to three essential oils that you enjoy. I have included my three staple essential oils for balancing mood and promoting a restful night's sleep.

YIELD: 1 application

1 cup sea salt

1 cup Epsom salt or magnesium flakes

½ cup baking soda

8 to 10 drops Relax and Restore Bath Blend, or essential oils of your choice (suggested oils: frankincense, lavender, clary sage, ylang ylang, or cedarwood)

RELAX AND RESTORE BATH BLEND

YIELD: 1 application

3 drops lavender essential oil

3 drops frankincense essential oil

2 drops clary sage essential oil

DIRECTIONS: Fill your bathtub with the hottest water you can stand. Mix together sea salt, Epsom salt, and baking soda in a small bowl. Add to the bath water. Blend essential oils together and add them to the bath.

Stir ingredients with your hands. Soak in the bath for 20 minutes and rinse off in the shower. Soak any longer and your body may reabsorb the toxins you have released. Rinse off the remaining salt on your body in the shower. While showering, visualize the water washing away all mental chatter and stress of the day.

Lather Up

Once you finish your therapeutic bath, finish the ritual off by indulging your skin with healthy, moisturizing oils. As you know, what you put on your skin enters your bloodstream. I recommend a shea butter and coconut oil blend to keep your skin moisturized and radiant throughout the year. For deep skin nourishment, apply this easy-to-make body butter recipe, or try the Homemade Citrus Body Butter found on page 123.

HOMEMADE CALMING BODY BUTTER

YIELD: 12-ounce glass container

1 cup unrefined shea butter

½ cup coconut oil

½ cup almond oil (or other carrier oil)

20 drops lavender essential oil

10 drops geranium essential oil

DIRECTIONS: Heat shea butter, coconut oil, and almond oil together over a double boiler. Cool mixture to room temperature. Add essential oils. Next, refrigerate mixture for an hour or so. Once solid, whip with mixing beaters until smooth. Store in a glass or stainless steel container.

Other suggestions for a 5-minute self-love ritual after the therapeutic bath:

🌿 A scalp massage with lavender and rosemary promotes relaxation, memory, and healthy hair. Combine these essential oils with coconut or avocado oil for a nourishing oil treatment.

🌿 Self-love massage with almond oil/coconut oil and your favorite muscle-soothing essential oils: white fir, lavender, cypress, wintergreen, or frankincense. Focus this self-massage on the neck, trapezius muscles, temples, shoulders, and let the tension of your day melt away.

The Mirror Exercise

I learned this ritual from a good friend, Tiffany Peterson, a year ago, and I practice this ritual each night, even when I am not feeling very worthwhile and joyful. I know that a lot of moms go to bed holding onto worries and feelings of unworthiness. These feelings can be difficult to shake and can wear down on our souls. I love this evening ritual right before bed to really conclude each day with abundance, appreciation, and love. This three-minute exercise is a very powerful and transformative experience. I recommend trying it out for 30 days to experience some incredible changes in your mindset. I think you will be pleasantly surprised by the results.

🌿 Find a mirror in your home, such as the bathroom or bedroom mirror. You will want to find a private space for this ritual. The purpose is to make eye contact with yourself in the mirror.

🌿 The first thing you will do is acknowledge your wins and accomplishments for the day. These can be small and big wins. Each day you make miracles happen for your family. Take a moment and own those wins.

🌿 After you have acknowledged your wins, you are going to declare your affirmations. I included some core affirmations below to incorporate, but feel free to create your own affirmations that are true for you and your life.

🌿 Lastly, this ritual ends with saying to yourself, "I love you."

Feel free to make the mirror exercise more transformative by incorporating essential oils before you begin. Essential oils that are beautiful for elevating this ritual are jasmine, frankincense, bergamot, melissa, and ylang ylang. I included a mirror ritual blend that has worked wonders for me.

AFFIRMATIONS:

I am enough.

I am beautiful.

I am worthy and deserving.

I am a loving and incredible mom.

I trust myself.

I allow myself the abundance I desire.

I am a miracle worker.

I am strong.

I am a powerful manifestor.

I was born to create my dreams.

I am overflowing with joy.

I radiate beauty, love, and grace.

MIRROR RITUAL ABUNDANCE BLEND

YIELD: 1 application

1 drop clary sage

1 drop lavender

1 drop bergamot

Setting the Mood for Sleep

The nightly ritual in my home involves using our essential oil diffusers to help everyone in the house wind down. There are so many wonderful calming blends that you can create, depending on the mood you want everyone to experience.

As you are heading to bed, here are a couple of rules for preparing for a good night's sleep. Put away electronics about an hour before bed and either have a nice conversation or read a book before turning in. Apply oils to your sheets and pillows with a spray bottle, and set the lighting to dim so that your sensory system is prepared for sleep. I recommend applying oils to the back of the neck, wrists, and bottoms of feet. Great oils for a restful night's sleep are cedarwood, clary sage, vetiver, and lavender. Choose one to two essential oils, apply to your palms, and take in three deep belly breaths, or diffuse them by your bedside while you are falling asleep.

SLEEP DIFFUSER BLEND

YIELD: 1 application

3 drops lavender

3 drop cedarwood

Alternate Nostril Breathing Ritual

We all know the importance of breathing. When you are under stress, breathing is the first thing to become shallow and strained. I encourage all types of breath work, because breath is capable of purifying the body and its seven energy centers, or chakras, giving movement to energetic blockages or within the body. One of my favorite breathing practices is Alternate Nostril Breathing. This really incredible two-minute Ayurvedic meditation technique is very powerful at reducing stress levels instantly. I recommend using calming essential oils to increase the effectiveness of this meditation. Try bergamot, frankincense, or clary sage.

DIRECTIONS: Start sitting in a cross-legged position facing east or north. Apply a calming essential oil like lavender or clary sage to your palms. Exhale all air. Close the right nostril with the right thumb, and inhale slowly and deeply into the belly through the left nostril. Pause. Close the left nostril with the ring finger, release the thumb, and slowly exhale through the right nostril. At the end of the exhalation, inhale through the right nostril, then close it with the thumb and exhale through the left nostril. This creates one round.

Begin with two rounds and gradually increase to 10.

CHAPTER

❦ 9 ❦

WOMEN'S HORMONE HEALTH AND ESSENTIAL OILS

Nowadays we are all overworked, which leaves no personal time or moments for reflection. This causes problems with energy as well as mood and cognitive management. And let's be honest, when we don't create balance in our day with simple, healthy habits and rituals, our hormones and health suffer. I can personally relate to feeling overworked and placing my health on the back burner for more demanding "priorities."

For many years now, I have heard from thousands of smart moms that something's just not right. They're sleeping less, feeling frazzled, and stress has become the default mode—even when life seems okay. They simply don't feel at home in their bodies the way they used to and are looking to move the needle with solutions that will have them feeling great again. Sound familiar?

Most of the women I run across have similar complaints, and while the concerns may vary, a common denominator exists—hormone chaos. The tricky thing about hormonal imbalance is that it often sneaks around in the background, wreaking havoc on your health before you even know it's there. Often women mistake irritability, sleeplessness, cravings, and mood changes as normal, or par for the course of being a busy mom. In our present-day culture, some of us even wear these warning signs as a badge of honor.

Understanding women's hormone health became a focus for me because I grew up in hormone chaos. I come from a lineage of women who struggle with hormones, starting with my mother's mother. Growing up, I didn't understand that it was hormones that had such an impact on my mom's health and happiness. Over the last several years, my mom struggled with perimenopause and menopause. While these are normal stages for women, the hormonal fluctuations can cause health concerns. There were many moments when she did not feel at home in her own body. Weight gain, sleeplessness, and mood swings were just some of the issues she experienced.

After many years of hormone struggles, my mom decided that implementing daily self-care habits, nutrition, supplementation, essential oils, and exercise was necessary for supporting her body and getting back the energy she desired. Many of the daily health habits and recipes featured in this chapter were implemented by my mom with strong conviction. Over the course of six months she lost 35 pounds, experienced more restful sleep, and had a more stable mood throughout the day. She also gained more energy and claimed she felt better than when she was in her twenties. She is a great example of how lifestyle, paired with plant-based nutrition and essential oils, is the key to a happy, balanced body.

By reading this chapter, you are taking the first step in creating hormone synergy within your body. You're joining a powerful community of smart moms who are committed to feeling amazing at every age! You deserve a body that works for you, and I am excited to share with you my favorite natural solutions to creating a body that you love. Now, it took me a while to realize how important it was to establish easy daily habits and rituals to get my body back on track and to release some of that overwhelm I was holding on to each day. I have been perfecting essential oil recipes for many years now, and I want to share in this chapter the main areas that most women want to work on when it comes to women's hormone health. I am going to share recipes for energy, cravings, emotional and mood support, sleep, stress, libido, and weight challenges. These essential oil recipes are designed to bridge the gap to healthy lifestyle changes that you can easily implement throughout the day. I believe that simple daily habits set the tone for the body you desire; they are the foundation for creating powerful transformations and results.

Stress Management

Is stress the culprit to hormonal imbalance in your body? It was the key component to my hormonal imbalance for many years. Stress has always been my Achilles heel, and in my mid-twenties I experienced a significant health crisis right in the middle of working on my doctorate, holding down a job to pay my mortgage, and taking on too many "other" priorities. My body hit a wall and I paid dearly for it.

Like many women that I know, I was determined to prove my worth through hard work, multitasking, and adding more to my plate. At some point my plate become a huge platter, and yet I still found myself stressing about not doing enough, especially for other people.

I remember the moment clearly; I was not myself anymore. I felt like a robot simply going through the motions—until I took a deep look into the decisions I'd made about my health, lifestyle, and happiness. Ultimately, I'd neglected myself over other pressing priorities. My constant "rushing" took a front seat to my health and my hormones suffered the consequences. In hindsight, I was suffering from Rushing Woman's Syndrome and it was wrecking my health and life! Rushing Woman's Syndrome was coined by Dr. Libby Weaver, and it describes the biochemical and emotional effects of constantly being in a rush and the health repercussions that urgency creates.

When I began to understand the physical and biochemical implications of rushing and stress wreaking havoc on my body, I realized that I wasn't the only woman suffering from these issues. Everywhere I looked, I met women with similar demands and countless priorities. These priorities were rarely centered around health until it was too late. As a practitioner, I have taken care of thousands of women dealing with a lack of energy, anxiousness, hormonal imbalance, weight gain, and chronic stress.

In a nutshell, constantly rushing from one priority to the next creates chronic stress in the body. This stress can affect nearly every physiological system in the body, from digestion to immunity. When reacting to stressors, the adrenal glands release hormones such as cortisol and epinephrine, which activate the sympathetic nervous system, also known as "fight or flight" response. This automatic fight-or-flight activation triggers the chain reaction of various organ systems to prepare for survival and protects us from sudden danger, like a tiger attack. Unfortunately, frequent activation of the sympathetic nervous system due to emotional, mental, and physical stressors can have extreme effects on our bodies over time, especially hormones in a women's body.

And, it's not just the physical health consequences that concern me when it comes to women. It's that they can live their lives so out of touch from their intuitions and passions, just like I experienced for many years.

Although I advocate hormone testing to figure out exactly what is going on in your body, there are key indicators to assess if your body is out of balance due to chronic stress. Below are some examples of what being out of balance can feel like on a daily basis:

- Your hormones are completely out of whack.
- You don't feel focused.
- You are exhausted in the middle of the day or morning.
- You are experiencing digestive issues (there is a connection between the brain and gut).
- You frequently experience head and neck tension.

- ❧ You are unable to lose weight.
- ❧ You are sick three to five times a year.
- ❧ You can't fall asleep at night due to mental chatter.
- ❧ You feel anxious and overwhelmed by your to-do list.
- ❧ You say things like: "I am crazy busy, I am in a rush, I've got to go, I am so tired."
- ❧ You don't remember how to feel calm and grounded.
- ❧ You don't feel happy and fulfilled.

If you can connect with two or more of these examples, I have some stress-busting strategies that will help move the needle toward hormonal harmony with ease and grace.

The first step to reducing stress in your life on a daily basis is to develop some self-awareness. Begin noticing those moments when you feel overwhelmed or rushed, and take a moment to reset your mental outlook of the situation. The more you begin to recognize when you are in a stressful situation, the more empowered you will be to choose a way out of those moments.

The next step to reducing stress is having a toolset on hand for those moments when you need to reduce stress and overwhelm. Essential oils are my favorite go-to natural solution for reducing stress and balancing mood. Aromatherapy is a powerful and effective solution for calming the mind and body. It's no surprise that essential oils are used in spa, meditation, classrooms, and healing facilities around the world to promote feelings of tranquility and calm.

As I mentioned in Chapter 7, research has demonstrated that simply inhaling the chemical constituents of an essential oil, or blend of essential oils, can elicit emotional responses and even promote emotional releases. Essential oils are some of nature's most powerful solutions for emotional health. Different essential oil aromas will elicit a different emotional response, individualized to each person. I welcome you to explore various essential oils and essential oil blends for those stressful moments when you need an instant mood reset. Below I am going to share some of my most practical and effective solutions for reducing stress and supporting mood management. These simple solutions and lifestyle techniques can be paired with the recipe blends below. The blends are designed to reduce feelings of stress, overwhelm, fearfulness, irritation, and other negative emotions. I want to point out that Chapter 8 is also a great resource to support your healthy, happy body.

Here are few effective solutions for reducing daily stress using essential oils:

- Begin a yoga practice 15 to 45 minutes per day, two to three days a week. Use lavender, bergamot, or the Calming Meditation Blend (page 146) while practicing your yoga.

- Practice mindfulness and meditation daily with wild orange essential oil or the Abundance Blend (page 147).

- Learn to let go of what does not serve you emotionally and physically. Become more aware of those times when you inadvertently let stress in. Clary sage is an ideal essential oil to keep on hand for these such moments.

- Reduce the stress in your body by consuming foods that support healthy gut health.

- Cleanse your body of unwanted toxins that lead to anxiety. Essential oils for purifying the body are lemon, grapefruit, and juniper berry. Reduce your toxic load by using the recipes in Chapter 5 and Chapter 6.

- Use essential oils aromatically. A diffuser is a good way to maintain a consistent level of therapeutic aromatherapy. Find my favorite aromatherapy blends in Chapter 7.

- Perform the Alternate Nostril Breathing Ritual on page 171. This technique is an effective way to allow your brain to go into neutral and take a relaxing pause from daily routine.

Stress Support and Mood Management Blends

OVERWHELM BE GONE

This is a powerful mood-reset blend. It's effective at releasing stress, balancing mood, and releasing tense emotions. This blend is also known to reduce irritable feelings throughout the day.

YIELD: 10-mililiter rollerball bottle

10 drops lavender essential oil

10 drops bergamot essential oil

7 drops clary sage essential oil

4 drops wild orange essential oil

2 teaspoons carrier oil of choice

DIRECTIONS: Add essential oils to the rollerball bottle and top off blend with a carrier oil of your choice. Apply to the back of neck, temples, wrists, mastoids, and behind the ears.

EMOTIONAL RELEASE DIFFUSER BLEND

This blend is ideal to add to a diffuser when you walk in the door from a long day or while at the office. You can also add 1 drop of each oil to your hands and take three deep breaths to release emotional distress. Geranium supports the release of unwanted emotions. Bergamot and jasmine stabilize mood and promote feelings of calm.

YIELD: 1 application

2 drops geranium essential oil

2 drops bergamot essential oil

2 drops jasmine or ylang ylang essential oil

DIRECTIONS: Add essential oils drops to an ultrasonic cool-air diffuser. If using a cool-air nebulizing diffuser, multiply this blend by 10 in a 15-milliliter glass bottle and run for 30 minutes to 1 hour before going to bed.

STRESS-FREE SPRAY

A stress spray is very easy to use during those moments when you are feeling overwhelmed. Lavender aids in relaxation and reducing tension. Wild orange and spikenard promote feelings of well-being and happiness, and peppermint invigorates the senses, helping to release worries.

YIELD: 2-ounce spray bottle

1½ ounces distilled water

10 drops wild orange essential oil

8 drops lavender essential oil

4 drops spikenard essential oil

4 drops peppermint essential oil

DIRECTIONS: Add water to spray bottle. Add essential oils, shake, and spritz. Spray blend in the car, into the air, and onto your body to melt stress away.

STRESS RELEASE RUB

Lavender and peppermint will ease tense muscles and clary sage is ideal for balancing mood.

YIELD: 1 application

2 drops lavender essential oil

2 drops clary sage essential oil

2 drops peppermint essential oil

1 teaspoon carrier oil of choice

DIRECTIONS: Combine essential oils with carrier oil of your choice, then massage 3 to 4 drops of blend into your shoulder, temples, back of neck, and wrists. Apply 1 to 2 drops to palms and breathe deeply to reduce stressful feelings. Use when needed.

Energy Support

"I just need more energy!" is a phrase that I hear a lot. A lack of sustainable energy is one of the biggest issues that women face today. Often, we show up as an empty vessel for those around us, especially ourselves. Unfortunately, coffee and sugar are not the solutions to this vicious energy-crashing cycle. One of the very first ways that I began to use essential oils was to experience an energy boost when I was feeling tired and overwhelmed. My go-to essential oil for months was wild orange. I called it my "energy bomb."

We know that essential oils with ketones and monoterpenes such as limonene and beta-pinene are incredible for uplifting mood and giving you the necessary energy boost that you need throughout the day. When it comes to using essential oils to achieve powerful results, it's important to understand that daily usage is very important. I use my energy rollerball blend two to three times a day, and sometimes more if I am working on a big project, traveling, or experiencing a really long day. These essential oil blends are very effective at delivering bursts of energy without the calories and caffeine.

INSTANT ENERGY BLEND

Wild orange and peppermint are my go-to energizer bunnies. Each of these essential oils are very versatile in supporting various functions of the body, but you will find that they are first and foremost energizing and awakening.

YIELD: 1 application

1 drop wild orange essential oil

1 drop peppermint essential oil

DIRECTIONS: Apply peppermint and wild orange essential oil to the palm, rub them together, and take 3 to 4 deep belly breaths. Repeat when needed.

ENERGIZER DIFFUSER BLEND

This is a family favorite in the house for getting things done with some zest and invigoration. This blend will encourage the entire family to push through any big task. This is also a perfect office blend. I typically diffuse this blend at the start of the morning to get everyone awake and moving, including myself.

YIELD: 1 application

2 drop lemon essential oil

2 drops grapefruit essential oil

1 drop spearmint or peppermint essential oil

DIRECTIONS: Add essential oils to a cold-water diffuser. If using a cool-air nebulizing diffuser, multiply this blend by 10 in a 15-milliliter glass bottle and run for 30 minutes to 1 hour, or apply 1 to 2 drops of blend to palms and take 3 to 5 deep belly breaths.

WAKE-UP MOMMA ROLLERBALL BLEND

Rollerball bottle blends are effective and efficient at providing a burst of energy. This blend combines eucalyptus and rosemary for supporting mental clarity. Peppermint and grapefruit are the ideal power combo for promoting alertness.

YIELD: 10-milliliter rollerball bottle

10 drops eucalyptus essential oil

10 drops rosemary essential oil

5 drops grapefruit essential oil

5 drops peppermint essential oil

Carrier oil of choice

DIRECTIONS: Add essential oils to rollerball bottle and top off blend with a carrier oil of your choice. Apply to the back of neck, wrists, temples, and back of ears.

MOTIVATION RESCUE ROLLERBALL BLEND

This blend is for those moments when you are feeling mentally and emotionally sluggish. Keep this blend in your purse for those midday slumps.

YIELD: 10-milliliter rollerball bottle

8 drops lime essential oil

8 drops rosemary essential oil

7 drops bergamot essential oil

5 drops basil essential oil

3 ylang ylang essential oil

2 teaspoons carrier oil of choice

DIRECTIONS: Add essential oils to the rollerball bottle and top off blend with a carrier oil of your choice. Apply to the back of neck, wrists, temples, and back of ears.

Sleep Support

Sleep is critical to our overall well-being and vitality, yet many moms sacrifice it or struggle getting enough sleep due to mental chatter, hormones fluctuations, and anxiousness. Not only are moms struggling to get enough sleep, they are also dealing with a lot of stress, which compounds over time and leads to hormone chaos.

The consequences of sleeplessness can be quite devastating to the body, especially the stress and sex hormones (cortisol, estrogen, and progesterone). Lack of sleep impairs judgment, concentration, and energy, and can lead to significant health issues over time. Currently, I know a lot of moms are either using sleep aids or wine to help them go to sleep at night. I would like to offer a more natural option that will work with your brain to promote tranquility and restful sleep throughout the night.

Although I addressed evening rituals in Chapter 8, I want to share with you some of my most effective sleep blends. The essential oils in these blends are made up of monoterpenes, sesquiterpenes, and alcohols, which are known to elicit feelings of tranquility and calm. These essential oils blends are not only great for mom, but they can be used for the entire family. My family has been using the essential oil sleep blends for over five years now and they continue to work effectively each night.

There are several ways that you can use these effective sleep blends. Nebulizing and ultrasonic cool-air diffusers are ideal for a restful night's sleep. I recommend adding your favorite essential oil sleep blend to the diffuser in the bedroom 30 minutes before bed. You can also use the sleep spritzer recipe below and spray your linens and pillows before going to bed. We keep a 2-ounce spray bottle by the bedside.

The last effective way to use essential oils to support tranquility and sleep is to apply a rollerball blend to the bottom of the feet, spine, and back of the neck 10 to 15 minutes or so before turning off the lights and falling asleep. Finally, add a couple drops to your hand and take three or five deep belly breaths right after you apply the oils topically.

The combination of aromatic and topical usage is ideal for reducing stress and mental chatter and promoting a good night's sleep. If you would like some other suggested sleep diffuser blends, I share a few more in Chapter 7.

The top 5 essential oils for tranquility and restful sleep are:

Cedarwood	Roman chamomile
Clary sage	Vetiver
Lavender	

SLEEPY-TIME SPRAY

Lavender and cedarwood are a powerful combination for a restful sleep. Other oils to incorporate are vetiver, bergamot, clary sage, and Roman chamomile.

YIELD: 2-ounce spray bottle

10 drops lavender essential oil

10 drops cedarwood essential oil

2 ounces distilled water or witch hazel

DIRECTIONS: Add water or witch hazel to spray bottle. Add essential oils, shake, and spritz. Spray Sleepy-Time Spray on pillows, comforters, and in the air before bed for a restful sleep.

SWEET DREAMS BLEND

This is a powerful sleep blend. It's effective at releasing stress, balancing mood, and promoting relaxation. This blend is also known to reduce anxious feelings throughout the day.

YIELD: 10-milliliter rollerball bottle

10 drops lavender essential oil

10 drops vetiver essential oil

7 drops marjoram essential oil

4 drops ylang ylang essential oil

2 teaspoons carrier oil of choice

DIRECTIONS: Add essential oils to the rollerball bottle and top off blend with a carrier oil of your choice. Apply to the back of neck, bottom of feet, and spine.

BEDTIME DIFFUSER BLEND

This blend is ideal to add to a diffuser for 30 minutes to 1 hour to unwind for a restful night. Cedarwood and clary sage are known as grounding essential oils. When combined with the sweetness of bergamot, this blend will get you ready for sleep.

Consider diffusing this blend 15 minutes before bed and continue to run it after you fall asleep.

YIELD: 1 application

2 drops clary sage essential oil

2 cedarwood essential oil

2 bergamot essential oil

DIRECTIONS: Add essential oils drops to a cold diffuser with water. If using a cool-air nebulizing diffuser, multiply this blend by 10 in a 15-milliliter glass bottle and run for 30 minutes to 1 hour before going to bed.

Cravings and Weight Challenges

Hormones can play a major role in increased cravings and stubborn weight gain. Stress, blood sugar imbalance, and thyroid and sex hormones all contribute to weight fluctuations. Our metabolism becomes sluggish, and food can become directly connected to our emotions.

Although I believe nutrition is the foundation to healthy hormone and weight changes, essential oils can bridge the gap for cravings and help to support a healthy metabolism. If you are interested in learning more about healthy recipes to support weight loss and stabilize blood sugar level, please check out two of my books: *The DASH Diet Cookbook* and *The Low-GI Slow Cooker*.

Essential oils can help control cravings and appetite, and promote healthy metabolism while increasing energy. My favorite way to use essential oils for this purpose is to breathe them in aromatically, or to add one to two drops of essential oils to my green smoothies or water infusions. The two water infusions that I use in this section can be found in my *Water Infusions* book.

When it comes to taking essential oils internally, you want to make sure your essential oils are safe for internal usage. As I explained in Chapter 2, not all essential oils are created equal and many cannot be internally ingested due to adulteration and synthetic chemicals. Please read the labels and do your research before adding essential oils to food and water.

CRAVING CONTROL BLEND

Peppermint and grapefruit are fantastic at reducing food cravings. Ginger and cinnamon add extra digestive and metabolic support.

YIELD: 10-milliliter glass container

20 drops grapefruit essential oil

10 drops peppermint essential oil

5 drops cinnamon essential oil

5 drops ginger essential oil

2 teaspoons carrier oil of choice

DIRECTIONS: Add essential oils to the glass container. Top off bottle with carrier oil and shake to completely blend essential oils. Apply 1 to 2 drops of blend to palms. Rub palms together and take 3 to 5 deep breaths to help reduce cravings.

SUGAR-BE-GONE BLEND

This blend is a lifesaver for anyone looking to avoid sugar during times when cravings are high. Breathing this blend is the best way to curb cravings and boost energy in a matter of minutes.

YIELD: 1 application

2 drops of peppermint essential oil

1 drop grapefruit essential oil

1 drop of lemon essential oil

DIRECTIONS: Add essential oils to a cold-water diffuser. If using a cool-air nebulizing diffuser, multiply this blend by 10 in a 15-milliliter glass bottle and run for 30 minutes to 1 hour, or apply 1 to 2 drops to palms and take 3 to 5 deep belly breaths for instant sugar craving support.

WEIGHT-LOSS POWER WATER

YIELD: 1 application

½ ruby red grapefruit, juiced

1 orange, juiced

2 Meyer lemons, 1 juiced and 1 sliced into wheels

1½ quarts still water

2 drops lemon essential oil

1 drop grapefruit essential oil

DIRECTIONS: Add the juices of the ruby red grapefruit, orange, and Meyer lemons to a small bowl. Pour juice through a fine-mesh sieve into a 2-quart pitcher. Add sliced lemon, cover with water, and then add essential oils. Refrigerate for at least 30 minutes, but preferably for 3 hours, before serving.

REFRESH AND RENEW

YIELD: 1 application

1 lemon, sliced into wheels

1½ quarts still water

2 drops lemon essential oil

1 drop peppermint essential oil

DIRECTIONS: Add lemon slices to the bottom of a 2-quart pitcher. Cover with water and add lemon and peppermint essential oils. Infuse for at least 30 minutes, but preferably for 2 to 3 hours, before serving.

DETOX BATH SOAK

Take a detox bath using the Cleansing Bath Blend once a month to support healthy metabolism.

YIELD: 1 application

1 cup sea salt

1 cup Epsom salt

½ cup baking soda

1 cup apple cider vinegar

1 application Cleansing Bath Blend

CLEANSING BATH BLEND

Rosemary, ginger, and grapefruit have purifying and cleansing properties and are great for your skin and digestive system.

YIELD: 1 application

5 drops rosemary essential oil

5 drops grapefruit essential oil

2 drops ginger essential oil

DIRECTIONS: Combine the sea salt, Epsom salt, and baking soda in a bowl. Combine all essential oils. Fill your bathtub with the hottest water you can stand. Add the dry ingredients, vinegar, and essential oils into the tub and mix with your hand. Soak in the detox bath for 20 minutes. Any longer, and your body may reabsorb the toxins you have released. Rinse off the remaining salt on your body in the shower.

Libido and Intimacy

Women want to know how to get their libido back. In my experience, the path to sexual energy is challenging for many women. Growing priorities and hormone changes lead to fatigue, overwhelm, and low libido. Very often, it seems like finding your libido takes more effort and energy than you have to give. Even though it may feel that way, I do think it's possible. I'm always looking for effective tools to support the emotional and physical component of libido, and essential oils are an ideal solution given their powerful, aromatic properties. By accessing the limbic brain through smell, essential oils can have a profound effect on libido and hormones.

Dr. Naresh Arora explains, "The essential oils do magic and stimulate the pituitary gland, the master of the endocrine gland, which controls hormone production. Inactiveness of pituitary gland can lead to low sex drive. So, the oils help keep it in an active state."

Essential oils and sensuality go hand in hand, and essential oils can increase interest in and enjoyment of sex and intimacy. While many essential oils are considered to have sensual properties, several emerge as the top sensual oils for women to promote sexual energy or libido: ylang ylang, bergamot, clary sage, rose, geranium, cinnamon, and sandalwood.

Essential oils can be used in a variety of ways that may enhance sensual feelings. Generally, these methods involve applying diluted essential oils to the skin, adding them to a bath, and inhaling the scent of the oils. Essential oils can be diluted in a carrier oil (such as almond oil, grapeseed oil, or fractionated coconut oil) and worn as a perfume throughout the day. The same essential oil blends can be used as a massage oil. In this section you will find recipes specifically created to boost libido and sensual emotions.

BLISSFUL NIGHT MASSAGE BLEND

The combination of cinnamon and sandalwood invigorates the senses and wild orange creates an intimate and uplifting mood.

YIELD: 1 application

5 drops sandalwood essential oil

5 drops wild orange essential oil

2 drops cinnamon essential oil

1 tablespoon carrier oil of choice

DIRECTIONS: Combine essential oils with carrier oil of your choice, then apply 10 drops of blend to the body for a blissful massage.

APHRODISIAC SPRAY

Sandalwood and geranium are known as sensual oils that elicit happy neurotransmitters. Ylang ylang and clary sage boost libido and support healthy hormone levels.

YIELD: 2-ounce spray bottle

1½ ounces distilled water essential oil

2 drops geranium essential oil

3 drops sandalwood essential oil

2 drops ylang ylang essential oil

3 drops clary sage essential oil

DIRECTIONS: Add water to spray bottle. Add essential oils in the spray bottle, shake, and spritz. Shake and spray on pillows, comforters, and in the air before bed to promote intimacy and sensuality.

SEDUCTIVE DIFFUSER BLEND

This blend is ideal to add to a diffuser 30 minutes to 1 hour before heading to bed to help get you in the mood for intimacy. This blend will also help to reduce stress and worry.

YIELD: 1 application

2 drops lavender essential oil

2 drops bergamot essential oil

1 drop ylang ylang essential oil

1 drop vetiver essential oil

DIRECTIONS: Add essential oils drops to a cold diffuser with water. If using a cool-air nebulizing diffuser, multiply this blend by 10 in a 15-milliliter glass bottle and run for 30 minutes to 1 hour before going to bed.

PASSION PERFUME BLEND

This blends carries many of the main aphrodisiac essential oils and smells incredible. This synergistic blend balances the nervous system and works on an emotional level to relax the senses, producing a feeling of optimism and euphoria. You can also make this into a massage oil.

YIELD: 10-milliliter rollerball bottle

10 drops sandalwood essential oil

10 drops ylang ylang essential oil

8 drops cinnamon essential oil

4 drops jasmine essential oil

2 teaspoons carrier oil of choice

DIRECTIONS: Add essential oils to the rollerball bottle and top off blend with a carrier oil of your choice. Apply to the back of the neck, spine, wrists, temples, and bottom of feet.

SENSUAL BATH SOAK RITUAL

YIELD: 1 application

BATH SOAK RECIPE

1 cup sea salt

1 cup Epsom salt

½ cup baking soda

SENSUAL BATH BLEND

4 drops lavender essential oil

4 drops ylang ylang essential oil

2 drops bergamot essential oil

1 drop vetiver essential oil

DIRECTIONS: Fill your bathtub with the warmest water you can stand. Mix together sea salt, Epsom salt, and baking soda in a small bowl. Add to the bath water. Blend essential oils together and add them to the bath. Stir the ingredients with your hands. Soak in the bath for 20 minutes, any longer and your body may reabsorb the toxins you have released. Rinse off the remaining salt on your body in the shower.

Note: This soaking ritual will get you in the mood for intimacy and love. The essential oils chosen in this blend help to uplift the mind and calm the senses. To accentuate your experience, consider using candle lights and soft music.

HOMEMADE SENSUAL BODY BUTTER

Once you complete your sensual bath soak, finish the ritual off by indulging your skin with a sensual essential oil body butter. This body butter can also be used for a massage.

YIELD: 12-ounce glass container

1 cup unrefined shea butter

½ cup coconut oil

½ cup almond oil (or any other oil)

5 drops sandalwood essential oil

5 drops ylang ylang essential oil

5 drops jasmine essential oil

DIRECTIONS: Heat shea butter, coconut oil, and almond oil together over a double boiler. Cool mixture to room temperature. Add essential oils. Next, refrigerate mixture for an hour or so. Once solid, whip with mixing beaters until smooth. Store in a glass or stainless steel container.

Perimenopause and Menopause

Let's be honest, hormones get blamed a lot, especially during perimenopause and menopause. It's very clear that hormones play a signification role in countless biochemical processes in the body, and when hormones begin to fluctuate, major shifts occur in the body that can feel uncomfortable and confusing.

The transition to menopause can be challenging physically and emotionally. Menopause is a very slow process, with perimenopause as the transitional phase. This transition can easily last more than five years. Most women begin to experience hormonal changes as early as 35 years old, but typically in their mid to late forties. On average, women reach menopause by 55 years old. Once a woman has experienced 12 months without a period, she is considered to be in menopause.

For each woman, the transition to menopause is different experience. Often, symptoms vary from person to person. In this chapter I've addressed many of the common hormonal concerns, but I would like to share a few more essential oil recipes that I have found very beneficial to women in this stage of transition. These essential oil recipes are designed to support physical and emotional hormone changes. I will be recommending ways that you can use essential oils topically and aromatically.

COOL YOUR HOT MESS SPRAY

Clary sage and geranium support healthy hormone function. Peppermint and lemon provide instant cooling relief.

YIELD: 2-ounce spray bottle

1½ ounces witch hazel

7 drops clary sage essential oil

5 drops geranium essential oil

5 drops peppermint essential oil

4 drops lemon essential oil

DIRECTIONS: Add witch hazel to the spray bottle. Add essential oils, shake, and spritz. Shake and spray on neck, chest, and anywhere that feels instantly overheated. Keep in your purse and use as needed.

COOLING PEPPERMINT CUCUMBER SPRITZER

Peppermint is very cooling on the skin and can be used to create a cooling sensation when instantly overheated. This spray is also wonderful after a workout or while outside in the sun. Avoid spraying blend into your eyes! Keep this spray in the refrigerator to last up to 2 months.

YIELD: 8-ounce spray bottle

1 Persian cucumber, peeled

2 teaspoons aloe vera

1 cup rose or clary sage hydrosol

10 drops peppermint essential oil

DIRECTIONS: Cut the Persian cucumber into chunks and blend with a blender or food processor until it's smooth. Strain this mixture through a cheesecloth or nut milk bag into a small clean bowl. Make sure to squeeze the cloth thoroughly to get all the liquid out. Add the rest of your ingredients and whisk well to make sure it's all blended together, then pour the liquid into a spray bottle. If the mixture is too viscous, just add more hydrosol or distilled water to dilute it.

THYROID SUPPORT BLEND

This blend is designed to support normal, healthy thyroid function. Clove and lemongrass have powerful antioxidant properties.

Frankincense, lemongrass, and myrrh promote healthy cellular function, and peppermint is stimulating.

YIELD: 10-milliliter rollerball bottle

10 drops frankincense essential oil

10 drops myrrh essential oil

8 drops lemongrass essential oil

4 drops clove essential oil

4 drops peppermint essential oil

2 teaspoons carrier oil of choice

DIRECTIONS: Add essential oils to the rollerball bottle and top off blend with a carrier oil of your choice. Apply to the thyroid, which is located on the throat, 2 times a day to support healthy thyroid function.

HORMONE SYNERGY BLEND

YIELD: 10-milliliter rollerball bottle

10 drops clary sage essential oil

8 drops lavender essential oil

8 drops geranium essential oil

4 drops bergamot essential oil

4 drops ylang ylang essential oil

fractionated coconut oil or almond oil

DIRECTIONS: Combine essential oils in a rollerball bottle, and then fill to the top with your carrier oil of choice. Roll the blends over your ovaries and pulse points (neck, ankles, and wrists) 2 to 3 times per day.

ADRENAL LOVE

Geranium and rosemary lessen stress and overwhelm. Clove contains powerful antioxidant support, and peppermint is stimulating and invigorating. This blend promotes healthy adrenal support.

YIELD: 10-milliliter rollerball bottle

8 drops geranium essential oil

7 drops rosemary essential oil

5 drops clove essential oil

2 drops peppermint essential oil

2 teaspoons fractionated coconut oil or almond oil

DIRECTIONS: Place the essential oil in a rollerball bottle, and then fill to the top with your carrier oil of choice. Roll the blends over your kidneys, located on the lower spine, morning and evening.

BRAIN FOG AND MEMORY BLEND

Frankincense and patchouli support focus, alertness, and healthy brain function. Lime and ylang ylang invigorate and support the emotional components of reasoning, planning, and problem solving.

YIELD: 1 application

10 drops frankincense essential oil

6 drops lime essential oil

6 drops patchouli essential oil

3 drops ylang ylang essential oil

1 tablespoon carrier oil of choice

DIRECTIONS: Combine essential oils with carrier oil of your choice; then, massage 3 to 4 drops of blend into bottom of feet, temples, back of neck, and wrists. Apply 1 to 2 drops to palms and breathe deeply to stimulate alertness and focus. Use when needed.

APPENDIX

ESSENTIAL OILS AT A GLANCE

ESSENTIAL OIL	TRAITS
Basil	Reduces tension; increases feelings of motivation and confidence; reduces muscle cramps when used in massage; provides sense of focus and mental clarity
Bergamot	Uplifting and calming; purifies and cleanses skin; eases digestive discomfort; relaxes stress and muscle tension
Cardamom	Provides relief from digestive upset; supports healthy respiration; soothing; enables mental clarity and openness
Cedarwood	Insect repelling properties; reduces nervousness; relieves respiratory discomfort; supports clear complexion
Cinnamon	Promotes oral hygiene; strengthens immunity; supports healthy metabolism and digestive function
Clary sage	Calming and relaxing; supports hormonal balance in women; soothes skin irritation; promotes restful sleep
Clove	Promotes oral hygiene; acts as insect repellent; supports immunity by providing antioxidants
Cypress	Emotionally grounding; reduces anxiety; rejuvenates and cleanses skin; tones complexion
Eucalyptus	Supports respiration and clear complexion; supports oral hygiene; reduces muscle tension; purifies air
Fennel	Supports healthy digestion and respiration; boosts metabolism; may reduce hunger and cravings
Frankincense	Promotes respiration and healthy inflammatory response; aids emotional and spiritual wellness; rejuvenates skin
Geranium	Soothes complexion; decreases stress; reduces appearance of skin blemishes; acts as insect repellent
Ginger	Eases occasional nausea and digestive discomfort; provides antioxidants; reduces bloating, gas, and indigestion
Grapefruit	Uplifting, balancing, and motivating; purifies air and hard surfaces; promotes clear, healthy skin; supports metabolic and digestive health
Helichrysum	Supports clear complexion; promotes regeneration of healthy skin cells; aids emotional and spiritual wellness; fades appearance of stretch marks, age spots, and other skin blemishes

Juniper berry	Purifies air; lessons stress and anxiety; supports mental clarity and healthy brain function; promotes feelings of positivity; detoxifying
Lavender	Soothes skin irritation; promotes restful sleep; supports cardiovascular system; reduces anxiety; boosts immunity
Lemon	Invigorating; purifying; provides powerful antioxidant properties
Lemongrass	Skin purifying; heightens awareness and promotes positive outlook; soothes muscles after exertion when used in massage
Lime	Energizing and uplifting; purifies air and hard surfaces; supports respiration; enhances complexion
Marjoram	Promotes restful sleep; supports cardiovascular and immune systems; provides emotional and spiritual balance
Melaleuca	Supports immunity; sooths skin irritation; cleanses and rejuvenates skin; purifies air and hard surfaces
Myrrh	Promotes healthy cellular function; provides mental clarity and focus; supports immunity; enhances emotional and spiritual balance
Oregano	Provides immune and digestive support; promotes healthy respiratory function; enhances cleaning products
Patchouli	Supports mental focus and healthy brain function; reduces appearance of blemishes; grounding and balancing
Peppermint	Supports respiration; promotes oral hygiene; alleviates stomach discomfort; promotes focus; soothes muscle aches
Roman chamomile	Calming; supports restful sleep; aids emotional and spiritual wellness; soothes skin irritation; eases discomfort from growing pains
Rosemary	Promotes healthy digestion and internal organ function; supports healthy hair; eliminates occasional fatigue; stimulating; may aid memory and concentration
Sandalwood	Supports restful sleep; promotes relaxation; reduces appearance of skin imperfections; balances emotions while lessening tension
Spearmint	Supports healthy digestion; promotes oral hygiene; uplifting, focuses the mind
Spikenard	Promotes feelings of well-being and happiness; uplifting; purifies skin and complexion
Vetiver	Supports restful sleep; calming, grounding, and relaxing
Wild orange	Simulating and uplifting; supports immunity and digestion; purifies air; good for cleaning and odor removal
Wintergreen	Promotes oral hygiene; eases muscle and joint pain
Ylang ylang	Aids emotional and spiritual wellness; nourishes skin; reduces stress and anxiety; supports restful sleep

BIBLIOGRAPHY

Althea Press. *Essential Oils for Beginners: The Guide to Get Started with Essential Oils and Aromatherapy*. Berkeley, CA: Althea Press, 2013.

Althea Press. *Essential Oils Natural Remedies: The Complete A-Z Reference of Essential Oils for Health and Healing*. Berkeley, CA: Althea Press, 2015.

AromaTools. *Modern Essentials, A Contemporary Guide to the Therapeutic Use of Essential Oils*. 5th ed. Orem, UT: AromaTools, 2013.

Barr, D. B., M. J. Silva, K. Kato, J. A. Reidy, N. A. Malek, D. Hurtz, M. Sadowski, L. L. Needham, and A. M. Calafat. "Assessing Human Exposure to Phthalates Using Monoesters and Their Oxidized Metabolites as Biomarkers." *Environmental Health Perspective*, vol. 111, no. 9 (July 2003): 1148–51, ncbi.nlm.nih.gov/pubmed/12842765.

Barr, L., G. Metaxas, C. A. J. Harbach, L. A. Savoy, and P. D. Darbre. "Measurements of Paraben Concentrations in Human Breast Tissue at Serial Locations across the Breast from Axilla to Sternum." *Journal of Applied Toxicology*, vol. 32, no. 3 (March 2012) 219–32, DOI: 10.1002/jat.178.

Barrett, Julia R. "Chemical Exposures: The Ugly Side of Beauty Products." *Environmental Health Perspectives*, vol. 113, no. 1 (January 2005): A24, ncbi.nlm.nih.gov/pmc/articles/PMC1253722.

Bronaugh, R. L., R. C. Wester, D. Bucks, H. I. Maibach, and R. Sarason. "In Vivo Percutaneous Absorption of Fragrance Ingredients in Rhesus Monkeys and Humans." *Food and Chemical Toxicology*, vol. 28, no. 5 (1990) 369–73, DOI: 10.1016/0278- 6915(90)90111-y.

dōTERRA. "The Blog Products." Accessed September 2, 2016. doterra.com/US/en/blog-products.

dōTERRA. "Essential Oil Application: Dilute or Not to Dilute." *dōTERRA Living Magazine* (Fall 2015). Accessed September 6, 2016. doterra.com/US/en/brochures-magazine-doterra-living-fall-2015-essential-oil-topical-application.

Environmental Working Group. *EWG's Skin Deep Cosmetics Database.* Accessed September 15, 2016. ewg.com/skindeep.

Fowler, P. A., M. Bellingham, K. D. Sinclair, N. P. Evans, P. Pocar, B. Fischer, K. Schaedlich, J. S. Schmidt, M. R. Amezaga, S. Bhattacharya, S. M. Rhind, and P. J. O'Shaughnessy. "Impact of Endocrine-Disrupting Compounds (EDCs) on Female Reproductive Health." *Molecular and Cellular Endocrinology*, Vol. 2 (May 2012): 231-239, ncbi.nlm.nih.gov/pubmed/22061620.

Fritz, Stephanie. "Are Oils Safe for Pregnancy and Breastfeeding?" *The Essential Midwife*. Accessed September 15, 2016. theessentialmidwife.com/oils-safe-pregnancy-breastfeeding.

Gillerman, Hope. *Essential Oils Every Day: Rituals and Remedies for Healing, Happiness, and Beauty*. San Francisco: HarperElixir, 2016.

Group, Dr. Edward. "3 Ways Endocrine Disruptors Destroy Your Health." *Global Healing Center*, 2015. Accessed September 15, 2016. globalhealingcenter.com/natural-health/3-ways-endocrine-disruptors-destroy-health.

Hill, Dr. David. "Ask Dr. Hill—Winter 2014." dōTERRA Blog. Accessed September 14, 2016. doterra.com/US/en/blog/healthy-living-ask-dr-hill-winter-2014.

Hill, Dr. David. "The Power of Aroma." *dōTERRA Living Magazine*. Spring 2015. Accessed September 13, 2016. doterra.com/US/en/brochures-magazines-doterra-living-spring-2015-the-power-of-aroma.

Hill, Dr. David. "The Value of Daily Use." dōTERRA Blog. Accessed September 28, 2016. doterra.com/US/en/blog/healthy-living-the-value-of-daily-use.

Keville, Kathi and Mindy Green. *Aromatherapy: A Complete Guide to the Healing Art*. 2nd ed. Berkeley, CA: Crossing Press, 2008.

Meeker, John D. "Exposure to Environmental Endocrine Disruptors and Child Development." *Archives of Pediatrics and Adolescent Medicine*, vol. 166, no. 1 (2012): E1-E7. ncbi.nlm.nih.gov/pmc/articles/PMC3572204.

Mercola, Dr. Joseph. "Is Your Perfume Poison?" Accessed October 3, 2016. articles.mercola.com/sites/articles/archive/2013/11/27/toxic-perfume-chemicals.aspx.s

Mercola, Dr. Joseph. "Women Put an Average of 168 Chemicals on Their Bodies Daily." Accessed October 2, 2016. articles.mercola.com/sites/articles/archive/2015/05/13/toxic-chemicals-cosmetics.aspx.

Pappas, Dr. Robert. "Essential Oil Myths." Essential Oil University. Accessed September 25, 2016. essentialoils.org/news/eo_myths.

Pert, Candace B. *Molecules of Emotion: The Science Behind Mind-Body Medicine*. New York: Simon & Schuster, 1999.

Price, Shirley and Len Price. *Aromatherapy for Health Professionals*. 4th ed. London: Churchill Livingstone Elsevier, 2012.

Purcheon, Nerys and Lora Cantele. *The Complete Aromatherapy & Essential Oils Handbook for Everyday Wellness*. Toronto, Ontario Canada: Robert Rose, Inc., 2014.

"Risks and Uses of Essential Oils." Wellness Mama. Accessed September 5, 2016. wellnessmama.com/26519/risks-essential-oils.

"RMS Beauty." Beauty Truth. Accessed September 2, 2016. www.rms beauty.com/pages/beauty-truth.

Rodriguez, Damian, DHSc, MS. "Emotional Aromatherapy: Science Meets Chemistry." dōTERRA Blog. Accessed September 2, 2016. doterra.com/US/en/blog/science-wellness-emotional-aromatherapy-psychology-meets-chemistry.

Sarantis, Heather, M.S., O. V. Naidenko, Ph.D., S. Gray, M.S., J. Houlihan, and S. Malkan. "Not So Sexy: The Health Risks of Secret Chemicals in Fragrance." Campaign for Safe Cosmetics. May 2010. Accessed September 29, 2016. ewg.org/sites/default/files/report/SafeCosmetics_FragranceRpt.pdf.

Schnaubelt, Dr. Kurt. *The Healing Intelligence of Essential Oils: The Science of Advanced Aromatherapy*. Rochester, VT: Healing Arts Press, 2011.

Tisserand, Robert. "Interview with Lebron Allen." Accessed September 15, 2016. roberttisserand.com/2015/08/robert-tisserand-interviewed-on-ingestion-dilution-and-other-safety-issues.

"Topical Use of Essential Oils." *dōTERRA Living Magazine*. Spring 2015. Accessed September 16, 2016. doterra.com/US/en/brochures-magazines-living-spring-2015-topical-use-of-essential-oils.

Total Wellness Publishing. *The Essential Life*. 2nd ed. Fontana, CA: Total Wellness Publishing, 2015.

Washington University. "Earlier Menopause Linked to Everyday Chemical Exposures." Accessed October 1, 2016. *ScienceDaily*. sciencedaily.com/releases/2015/01/150128141417.htm.

Worwood, Valerie Ann. *The Complete Book of Essential Oils & Aromatherapy*. Novato, CA: New World Library, 1991.

Worwood, Valerie Ann. *The Fragrant Mind: Aromatherapy for Personality, Mind, Mood, and Emotion*. Novato, CA: New World Library, 1996.

INDEX

Note: Unless noted otherwise, throughout this index, "oils" refers to "essential oils."

ACKNOWLEDGMENTS

I want to acknowledge all of the smart, loving moms that inspired me to create this book and the recipes in it. I know that natural solutions are a priority for many moms around the world and I hope that you will find incredible solutions within these pages.

I also want to acknowledge the amazing tribe of women that I get to work with every day who change lives by sharing and educating about the benefits of essential oils. You are making a huge difference in this world, one drop at a time.

I want to thank Erin Hubbard for your continued recipe inspiration and collaboration on this incredible book. I couldn't have completed this without you.

To my amazing friends, colleagues, and family for supporting me and providing the right amount of advice while I wrote the book, and for sharing great ideas on how to get it out to the masses.

And lastly, I want to acknowledge my husband Alex for supporting me during those long days and nights testing recipes and writing the book. You are amazing and the best partner I could have on this incredible journey!

ABOUT THE AUTHOR

Dr. Mariza Snyder is a passionate wellness practitioner and public speaker with more than eight years of experience focusing on women's hormone and menopause health. Dr. Mariza leads a community of women who educate about nutrition, detox programs, self-care rituals and essential oils. She graduated Cum Laude from Life Chiropractic College West in 2008. She has a background in biochemistry and certifications in nutrition and aromatherapy.

Currently, Dr. Mariza serves as an educator on topics relating to women's hormone health. She's the creator of the Women's Balance Summit and author of five additional books: *The DASH Diet Cookbook*, *The Low-GI Slow Cooker*, *The Antioxidant Counter*, *Water Infusions*, and *The Matcha Miracle*. Check out her website, drmariza.com, for women's hormone and menopause tips, including recipes and remedies.